Contents

About the authors

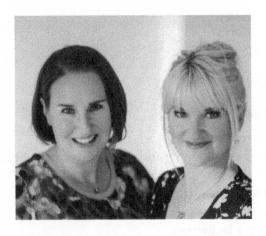

We are both practicing healthcare professionals with a combined clinical experience of over 45 years.

Karen graduated from the University of Cambridge Medical School. She is a GP in South Yorkshire, a GP trainer and GP appraiser. She also organizes and facilitates the ongoing continuing professional development of GPs in Doncaster. Since the beginning of her career, Karen has committed to working holistically, empowering her patients. Karen has also been a BBC Radio Leeds GP since 2005, volunteering her time to promote health education across the UK.

Chrissie is a charted physiotherapist, graduating from Sheffield Hallam University. She completed a diploma in Hypnotherapy and became a practitioner of NLP in 1998. Chrissie is a shamanic practitioner and reiki healer. She finished a diploma of psychotherapy and CBT in 2019. Chrissie runs her own holistic physiotherapy and sports therapy clinic. Chrissie is also a 'professional' for BBC Radio Leeds.

We are passionate about wellbeing, and we believe that personal resilience is the key. It is essential to enable and empower people to take responsibility for this. Our approach is a unique blend of spirit and science, combining our expert knowledge with the individual's expert knowledge of themselves.

We believe that *everyone* has the capacity for enormous growth. We offer interactive resilience training for all via our website <www.resilientpractice.co.uk>. We also teach for the Royal College of General Practitioners and Health Education England.

Foreword

'Resilience' is a word that often gets bandied about without any context. It refers to the ability to adapt or recover after a period of change or difficulty. It is a word we need to understand more now than ever before.

Periods of difficulty come in many forms: maybe in the changes the COVID-19 pandemic has thrown at us, the way we perceive ourselves, the way we feel about ourselves, our physical health, the way other people make us feel, or the way the world around us makes us feel. Our mental health is affected by all of these things.

None of us are successful all the time; recognizing how to turn our struggles into positive experiences that we can learn from is key, and this book will help you do just that.

Dr Karen Forshaw is a holistic medical practitioner and Chrissie Mowbray is a physiotherapist, hypnotherapist and psychotherapist. Together, they have over 45 years' experience in managing people's mental and physical health, and understand how intertwined the two are. They have drawn on their wealth of experience working with those who live with anxiety and stress every day and have come up with a book that allows the reader to recognize the issues that are holding them back. They explain the science behind why we feel the way we do, using modern medicine and ancient wisdoms passed down through a variety of cultures.

Karen and Chrissie show us how to best manage those thoughts of self-doubt we all have, that stop us in our tracks, that little voice that tells we are not good enough, that feeling of 'imposter syndrome' that blights our biggest moves. More importantly, they offer simple pragmatic tips for how to tackle even the most difficult of situations.

One of the things I find hardest is saying 'no' to people. As my life has got busier, this has led to me spending less time doing the things I enjoy the most and more time people-pleasing. Reading this manual has helped me recognize what it was about me that made this difficult, what things had happened to shape my mind so much that I found it hard to say 'no'. Now I am better at prioritizing my family and myself and, importantly, have no guilt about it. On the days I am feeling overwhelmed, I now have several mindfulness techniques and breathing exercises that allow me to focus my mind and get on with the task at hand, not letting it overcome me.

This is a book for all us who have ever suffered from anxiety, stress or low self-esteem: it gives us the tools to break free from the shackles of these things and finally be free.

Dr Amir Khan

Introduction

> Do not judge me by my success, judge me by how many times I fell down and got back up again.
>
> *Nelson Mandela*

Hello. We are Dr Karen Forshaw and Chrissie Mowbray. *How to Rise: A Complete Resilience Manual* teaches wellbeing and resilience skills from a unique perspective. We are highly accomplished health professionals who emphatically recognize the power of spirit.

Throughout our careers we have journeyed through the philosophies of East and West. We have translated everything that we have learned into practical and accessible resilience tools for you. We will explain the scientific language of resilience and mental health, aligning it to the spiritual teachings threaded throughout all cultures.

In our many years of clinical experience, the most common symptom we have seen is anxiety. In fact, we believe that the majority of the population has a certain level of anxiety bubbling away under the surface. It becomes more apparent for everybody in stressful situations and when we are under pressure. Anxiety is also a symptom of many conditions relating to all sorts of conditions, issues and problems, including:

- depression
- stress
- low self-worth
- panic attacks
- trauma and abuse
- childhood trauma
- bereavement
- insomnia

- weight loss and body image
- IBS
- addiction
- relationship problems
- performance issues
- communication difficulties
- pain
- isolation

- debt
- gender
- sexuality.

This list is not exhaustive.

Chronic anxiety is a problem in itself. It can result from terrible trauma but can also be present with no apparent cause. In both cases it can lead to great suffering. We have seen many people in this situation. There are many who feel that their anxiety is unwarranted. This often leads to feelings of shame and guilt, which compounds the situation.

Those who suffer with chronic anxiety can start to believe that this is a part of who they are, predetermined and present in their blueprint.

Many years ago Chrissie was attending a 'Mind, Body and Spirit Fair'. She noticed a woman sitting quietly at a small, undecorated table. She was a healer. She was not selling anything; she was simply offering her wisdom with a bowl of cards. The healer pulled a card and directed Chrissie to recall a time when she had been held back by her need for approval. This prompted a deep conversation that culminated in Chrissie describing herself as an 'overthinker'. She had always considered this a root cause of her own anxiety and had accepted it as part of her make-up.

The healer's response to this struck her deeply. 'Stop saying that. Every time you say it, you drive it deeper. It is NOT who you are. It is just something you have been doing up until now.'

Chrissie left with a new perspective. It prompted her to do some inner work. She realized that overthinking was a *choice*.

Overthinking is most often negative and usually repetitive. It leads to anxiety. It is a behaviour that we can choose whether to engage in or not. This book will show you an alternative path.

A diagnosis of anxiety should prompt a deep dive into your psyche to examine where the negative, repetitive thought patterns are coming from. This book is that deep dive.

Each of us has experienced challenges in our personal and professional lives, and it is in working through those wounds, and helping our patients to do the same, that we have come to write this book. We have both suffered from chronic anxiety and feelings of low self-worth. Karen's mum was diagnosed with advanced cancer and that knocked Karen's ability to cope. This experience, and helping patients on a daily basis, is a conduit to her healing. Chrissie has been walking the path of meditation, mindfulness and healing since early adulthood.

We are alchemists who have transmuted our wounds into tools. In our book we share with you how to do the same.

How to navigate this book

The book is easy to navigate. It is set out in three functional parts: Theory, Core Skills and a Resilience Toolkit (an extensive list of practical tools with specific purposes).

In Part 1 we break resilience down into its component parts and show you how to measure your current resilience with our Resilience Gap Analysis Tool. This is a questionnaire designed to cover all aspects of wellbeing and shows you where, in your life learning, some resilience tools would be beneficial.

We then explore the self-awareness that is required to build resilience, translating Western psychology and Eastern philosophies into an accessible language for all. These chapters will encourage a deep understanding of self-awareness, allowing you to see that you alone are responsible for your wellbeing. Knowing this gives you power to change and helps you to identify what to work on.

Often, self-help books stop here; readers are left with the knowledge of where they need change but not how to make it happen.

This book is different.

Part 2 teaches a set of core skills, providing you with the basic techniques that you need to get the most from your

Resilience Toolkit. We have distilled these skills from both modern and ancient practices across the globe. They will help you to apply the knowledge of self-awareness that you gained in Part 1, and prepare you to use the tools in part three. Examples include observation, the removal of obstacles, basic breathing techniques, meditation skills, mindfulness, language and cultivating a resilient mind-set.

Part 3 contains a vast array of practical, cross-cultural tools and exercises from which you will create your own tailor-made 'Resilience Toolkit'. These include original meditations with specific purpose, visualization exercises, healthy rituals, organizational tools, reframing exercises, conflict resolution tools, physical exercises, NLP tools, manifestation techniques, grounding exercises, the Five-Point Rescue Plan and shamanic tools.

We have made these both practical and accessible in a 'how to' format. The tools are mapped to the individual reader's Resilience Gap Analysis using a key. Each question in the analysis has a designated number, and all the tools which are useful or helpful for that question are marked with that number. The tools are also mapped to common problems. These common problems have been designated with a letter, and the tools which will help in each situation are marked with that letter.

How to use this book

There are many ways to use this book. You can read it from start to finish, or you can jump straight to the tools and then back them up with the theory. You can learn a core skill that resonates with you, or you can approach the book with a specific problem and practise the tools that address your issue. The Resilience Gap Analysis Tool is a fantastic way to identify areas that need your attention. You can then select the appropriate skills and tools.

Self-awareness is the most empowering thing anyone can experience. Our mission is to pass this message on. We use our resilience tools and techniques on a daily basis; we also help our patients to do the same.

We look forward to working with you.

Chrissie and Karen

Part 1
THEORY

1

What is resilience?

Resilience can go an awful long way.

Eddie 'the Eagle' Edwards

Resilience

Resilience *(noun)*: The capacity to recover quickly from difficulties; the ability of a substance or object to spring back into shape.

Resilience is the ability to bounce back when things do not go the way that you had hoped. Being resilient does not magically make our difficulties disappear, but it allows us to see beyond them and get the best outcome from the current situation.

Often, we do not have control over things that happen and we can end up in situations where our ability to cope is sorely tested. When the environment becomes stormy, if our levels of resilience do not respond then we can become swamped.

If we have, at our fingertips, an array of tools and techniques to improve our resilience skills then we survive and, better than that, we thrive.

Resilience is synonymous with buoyancy, staying afloat whatever the condition of the surrounding seas. There is a school of thought that encouraging resilience in people is asking them to put up with toxic environments. We believe, however, that resilient people will go on to create kinder environments.

Many people decide that they are not resilient, and that they are powerless to do anything about it. We need to *wake up* to the fact that resilience is entirely within our control. This book will help you to do just that. We will help you to become self-aware and expand your toolbox of resilience skills – and you will *RISE!*

Understanding resilience

Human beings have adapted to live in all parts of the globe in a relatively short space of time. This is a sign of our innate resilience. Our levels of success are a product of our interactions with the environment; adverse events and environmental stressors are weighed against our resilience skills. Building our repertoire of resilience skills tips this scale in our favour, and we flourish.

To develop these skills, we first need to understand the components of resilience. The more we know about these components, the better able we are to make positive changes. In addition, we will discuss the importance of establishing a baseline measurement of resilience – this allows us to monitor our progress as we walk the path of enlightenment.

Resilience has been researched scientifically for decades. Over time it has been classified in different ways. In evaluating that research, we have identified four distinct components: *psychological* resilience, *emotional* resilience, *physical* resilience and *relationships*.

Psychological resilience

In observational studies of thousands of children, Norman Garmezy[1] identified that a child's ability to thrive was determined by both internal and external factors. He determined that some children flourished despite extreme social deprivation and a significant lack of parental support. He concluded that these children had innate characteristics that helped them thrive. This is 'resilience'.

Similarly, Emmy Werner[2] followed the lives of 698 children on a Hawaiian island. She saw that, despite some of the most adverse early life events, a significant proportion of the children developed into successful adults. A stable positive adult presence was important, but there were children who flourished without this. Those children who thrived despite a lack of early support demonstrated a strong sense of self-awareness. Werner talked about this in terms of the children's 'locus of control'. This term, first coined by Julian B. Rotter, describes how much a person believes they are in control of their own life; in other words, their degree of belief in their own ability to change their life rather than being at the mercy of external circumstances.

Those with a strong *internal* locus of control recognize that they have the power to control their lives via their own responses. Those with a strong *external* locus of control have given away their power and do not accept responsibility for what happens to them. The locus of control is, in fact, a spectrum and we all sit at some point along it. Our position on this spectrum can vary depending on our circumstances. For example, a traumatic event may lead to it becoming more external. Werner's study suggests that, the closer one sits to the internal end of the spectrum, the more resilient one is. The fact that this point can move means that it can be consciously changed.

The studies discussed above prove that those who have experienced adverse events in childhood can still be extremely resilient and experience success. A strong *internal* locus of control can thus make up for adverse events at any age.

To have an *external* locus of control is to tell yourself that you are powerless; you have no control over what happens in your life. Giving away responsibility for our thoughts and feelings disempowers us and leaves us vulnerable and less resilient.

In contrast, those with a strong internal locus of control recognize and own their own thoughts and feelings. They understand that others do not have the power to affect their emotions unless they choose to let them. If someone is rude, they are rude. *We* decide how to respond. We can choose whether it affects us or not. No one has the power to make us angry, upset or confrontational – unless we give it to them.

Being self-aware and developing a strong internal locus of control will clearly improve our resilience.

Emotional resilience

How we think or conceptualize things has a great impact on our resilience. Do we think in positive or negative ways? Is our cup half full or half empty?

We have little control over our childhood, our life experiences or our current environmental stressors. We do, however, have the ability to think about them in a different way. We can take control of how we perceive any life event. Any trauma can be seen as an opportunity. At the beginning of the twentieth century, Austrian psychologist Alfred Adler stated: 'We are not determined by our experiences, but by the meaning we give to those experiences.'[3]

More recently, George Bonanno[4] described that while we are all subject to the same evolutionary fight/flight mechanisms that served to protect our ancestors, our responses can be very different. We have the same rush of the stress hormones, adrenaline and cortisol, but some of us perceive events as trauma and others see them as opportunities for growth.

What they are both saying is that we can choose how an event affects us. We can give our power to it, calling it a trauma and feel all the negative emotions that go along with that. Alternatively, we can search for a positive aspect in the event. This might be an opportunity to right a wrong, a chance to learn a skill that will prevent a similar experience, or an opening to move towards a better future.

It is very important to stress that this is not about asking the sufferer of the trauma to take responsibility for what happened, nor is it condoning the action. This is about allowing the sufferer to take back their power in order to effect recovery.

Every event is an opportunity to learn about the Self and hone our resilience skills. We must learn to give meaning to adverse events in order to see them as opportunities. Choosing to see the positives in any given situation makes us more resilient and guides us safely through life.

Barbara Fredrickson's work further supports this. In her book *Positivity*,[5] the American psychologist describes how people with a positivity ratio of 3:1 (those who have three positive thoughts and feelings for each negative thought, over a period of time) 'flourish', while those who have a lower ratio 'languish'. Her 'broaden and build' model explores how the effects of positive thoughts and feelings may not be felt as instantly as negative ones, but are every bit as powerful. If you drop a vase, there is an instant effect: the event shocks you and immediate negative thinking follows, for example 'I'm so clumsy' or 'I'm so stupid'.

Positive actions, such as taking flowers to a sick relative, give a less intense feeling. The positive effects, however, accumulate over time. Fredrickson shows us that 'broadening' our self-awareness, encouraging new ideas and motivating us to try new things allow us to 'build' and develop skills, networks and supports, thereby improving our resilience.

Thinking in a positive way is something that we can learn to do.

Physical resilience

As healthcare professionals, we know that our overall resilience is affected by our health. In turn, our physical resilience is affected by the lifestyle choices we make. Adequate sleep, regular physical activity and a healthy diet have all been proven to contribute significantly to our wellbeing.

Poor sleep is a recognized symptom of anxiety and depression. Studies have also shown that poor sleep can contribute to the development of these conditions.

A lack of good-quality sleep has negative physical and psychological effects. Physically, our immune system is impaired, our blood pressure goes up, as does our risk of developing cardiovascular disease and diabetes. Psychologically, our memory, reaction time and performance are impaired and, as stated above, our risk of anxiety and depression are increased.[6]

The amygdala is the part of our brain that controls the fight/flight response caused by negative stimuli. When we are sleep deprived, our amygdala becomes overactive – initiating the fight/flight response following lower levels of stimulus, releasing stress hormones into our bodies. All of these factors impact on our ability to think positively and, therefore, affect our level of resilience.

Physical activity is known to disperse cortisol – a stress hormone. It also releases endorphins in our brain that make us feel happier and more positive. A 2015 study showed that regular exercise protected against the negative emotions common after an adverse event.[7]

Our diet can have profound effects on our physical and mental health. Direct effects include the irritability we feel from yo-yoing blood sugar levels (caused by eating high-sugar foods) and poor concentration caused by dehydration. Vitamins, minerals and proteins are essential for healthy cells. Caffeine is a stimulant, and too much can impair our functioning. Alcohol is an anxiolytic and is commonly used to wind down at the end of a hard day. Some may even think of it as one of their current resilience tools; however, it is a maladapted coping mechanism. Regular excessive alcohol consumption actually causes depression and impacts on the quality of our sleep.

The indirect effects of a poor diet include problems with body image, which commonly impact on feelings of self-worth and self-esteem. This moves us towards the external locus of control, which we know reduces our resilience.

Relationships and resilience

Hindu swamis, whose goal is spiritual transcendence, often live alone as hermits, cut off from the rest of the world. Ultimately, true resilience is being independent of anyone and unaffected by anything. For most of us, however, this is not real life. Human beings exist in multiple social groups, and we are supported by those networks. There is a difference between someone who *chooses* to be alone because they do not need connection, and someone who is *lonely* because they cannot make connections or they perceive that they need more connections than they currently have.

To be truly resilient, we should aim to detach from the need for connection but possess the skills required to connect should the need arise.

Our childhood, our life experiences and our social networks all contribute to our resilience. Our early life experiences are clearly important; a positive, loving adult role model gives a child the first building blocks of resilience. This was observed by Werner and her team in Hawaii. The adult did not need to be a parent – a sibling, a teacher, a coach or minister served in the same way.

Human cooperation first developed in our ancestors as a protective mechanism. In the harsh existence of primitive humans, anything that improved survival was worth cultivating. Social interaction was a big part of this. For modern humans the threats to survival are very different, but the need to make connections has remained and there are benefits to social networks. Research by Teo et al.[8] has shown that poor-quality social relationships are a risk factor for developing depression. Human studies have shown that people with poor social support have higher levels of stress hormones and they release these hormones to smaller stimuli than those with good relationships.

We can work to build our networks and make connections, thinking of these as our safety net, there to protect and support us when things go wrong. Fredrickson's broaden and build model, described above, shows how positivity helps develop these networks and how these networks support and help us to flourish.

Our social networks include all aspects of our life: our homes, places of education and our place of work. Talking to people who we know care about us is an important coping mechanism, and the ability to communicate with others is a resilience tool.

The number of relationships required to support one's resilience will be entirely individual. The key is to have people we can trust who provide a warm, loving environment when we need it. The ability to build these relationships is a skill that can be learned.

To summarize, our resilience is made up of multiple factors. We have varying degrees of influence over these factors. We can work towards moving our locus of control to be internal, we can develop our self-awareness, reframing our thoughts in a positive way, and we can make healthy lifestyle choices. We can acknowledge our early life experiences without letting them define us, and we can build our social networks to support us.

Throughout this book we will describe, in detail, how to build on these four key components of resilience.

In addition, breaking resilience down in this way allows us to measure our individual strengths and current needs. This then directs us to where we need to work.

Measuring resilience

Before we start to build our Resilience Toolkit, it is important to establish a baseline measurement of our current resilience. This will help us to track our progress on the path towards enlightenment.

Why do we measure anything? Measurements allow us to be accurate, rather than making assumptions about things. Also, paying attention to a measurement can help us to identify previously unrecognized patterns in our behaviour. Measuring allows us to identify key areas that require work. As humans, we are attracted to things that we are good at and we often avoid the things that need the most attention. This is because we have decided the solutions are too hard or not what we want to do. This is 'resistance' and will be explored, in detail, in the Core Skills section.

By measuring our resilience, we make sure that we spend our time building skills in the areas we need, not simply reinforcing our areas of already resilient practice.

In our experience, measurements are most valuable when they are made by the individual. Measures of attitudes, values and behaviours are subjective and, therefore, best made using questionnaires.

There have been many resilience scores published over the years. All are a series of questions that incorporate the author's construct of resilience. It is important, however, to remember that a score or measure of any kind is useful only if its purpose is clear.

We have devised a questionnaire that covers all the factors that influence resilience: purpose, autonomy, conflict, work–life balance, health, social support, organization and self-awareness.

You can download your Resilience Gap Analysis Tool from our website: www.resilientpractice.co.uk

If you prefer pen and paper, there is a printed copy at the end of the chapter.

Do not overthink the questions! Give your current score out of 10 and your ideal score, remembering that this might not be ten out of ten.

The purpose of the questionnaire is not to receive an overall resilience score but to highlight the areas where you perceive your resilience to be lower.

The questions with the largest gap between your current and ideal scores are the areas of your life which will benefit the most from you focusing on them. This is where learning some new resilience tools will be useful. Part 3 contains an extensive collection of tools. The tools have been mapped to the Gap Analysis showing which are likely to be useful for each question. This is, however, not fixed. It is important you find tools that resonate with you, as these are the ones that you will enjoy and which will work for you.

The power of the Resilience Gap Analysis Tool is that it is individual to you. Everyone will have different current scores, and, more importantly, they may have different ideal scores. For example, some people place less importance on support from peers than others.

A further power of the tool is that you can revisit the questionnaire whenever you want to. If you see a gap and try a new resilience tool, you can assess its effectiveness.

In conclusion, in this opening chapter, we have explored resilience to understand its multifaceted nature and we have addressed its measurement to recognize in which key areas we need to build our skills and to track our progress.

In the next chapters of the book, we will break down and examine the multiple components of self-awareness, giving you a deeper understanding and encouraging your spiritual evolution.

Being resilient does not mean never feeling down or upset. It is about allowing adverse events to test us – giving us the opportunity to use all the skills and tools we have amassed to come out on top.

Resilient practice: The Resilience Gap Analysis Tool

Please score yourself on the following questions as truthfully as you can. This questionnaire is for your own use to help you recognize which resilience skills you should include in your toolkit.

	Current (1–10)	Ideal (1–10)	Gap
How well do you manage your workload?			
How well do you cope with uncertainty?			
How much of your time do you spend ruminating about past/future events?			
How often do you find yourself absorbing the emotional distress felt by others?			
How often do you go home feeling significantly drained of energy?			
How much pressure do you put on yourself to achieve your goals? a. Professional b. Personal			
How do you rate your health habits in terms of a. Sleep? b. Physical activity? c. Diet?			
How do you rate your work–life balance (e.g., working late or at home)?			
How do you rate your organizational skills?			
How well do you manage your time?			

How well do you communicate with
  a. Family and friends?
  b. Colleagues?			

How well do you manage
inappropriate requests from
  a. Family and friends?
  b. Colleagues?			

How well do you process irritation
caused by
  a. Family and friends?
  b. Colleagues?			

How well do you adapt to change?			
How well do you cope when things go wrong?			
How well supported do you feel by your peers?			
How supportive are your social relationships?			
How comfortable are you in sharing experiences with peers?			
How well do you process feedback?			
How well do you manage conflict?			

Once you have established where your biggest gaps are, you can start looking for the tools which will help you the most.

You can re-evaluate your Gap Analysis whenever you like, to demonstrate quality improvement.

2

Exploring conditioning and uncovering core beliefs

Eventually, even Pavlov found that when he heard a bell, he had the overwhelming urge to feed a dog.

Julian K. Jarboe

In this chapter, we will explore how everything that has shaped you affects how you respond to everything that happens to you. It is, ultimately, about how human perspective affects human behaviour.

We all have our own unique model of the world. This is how we make sense of our lives and learn how to behave in order to survive.

Our model of the world is comprised of the following:

- information from our parenting
- information from life experiences and lessons
- genetic make-up.

The first two of these can be described as *conditioning*. This is the phenomenon where a person's reactions and responses to life events are created in childhood, through learning from the external environment.

It is from the above sources of information that we construct a set of core beliefs about the Self. These help us to understand who we are in order to interact in the world in safety.

Using both our positive and negative core beliefs and experience, we collect and implement behavioural traits, likes, dislikes and characteristics which can be described as *personality*.

This is who we *think* we are. Who we *actually* are, is everything that we were born with and pure, unbound *potential*.

When we are constrained by core beliefs and 'personality', we do not reach that full potential. This means that, if you do not like an aspect of your personality, or a deeply rooted pattern of behaviour, it can be changed.

It is widely accepted that our core beliefs drive our thoughts. These thoughts then drive our emotions. Emotions then lead to behaviour. If the thoughts and emotions are negative, they can lead to damaging repetitive behaviours, including further negative thinking. This is the CBT model.[1] Our tools aim to teach how to reframe those core beliefs and thought processes to effect positive change.

We will discuss this, in much more detail, as a core skill in Chapters 9 and 15.

Let us now explore how this information is presented to us in early life.

Parenting

The manner in which we were parented significantly influences our model of the world. We learn our basic survival skills from parents or carers. This is also our first experience in how to relate to other human beings.

In childhood, we strive to gain love, attention, affection and approval. Our survival depends on it. For a helpless child, survival is of paramount importance and can be assured only by learning the rules of interaction with the family members on whom they depend for their basic needs. Those rules will be unique to each household and form the beginnings of how a person understands relationships.

In childhood, we learn how to relate to others by observing the relationships of those who are close to us, and by interacting in relationships ourselves. Each child will collect a unique set of data, even children belonging to the same household. This is because they each have a unique genetic make-up and are born into a different position within the family. They may have similar experiences but will process them differently.

Parenting skills are learned from parents or carers when we are children. This means that unhealthy or unwanted patterns of behaviour can be passed down through subsequent generations. In shamanism, we talk about ancestral healing. This is where we examine and work with harmful, inherited behaviour patterns which we feel have been carried down through our family in a way which affects us negatively in the present. We can translate this by explaining that we learn from our own parents, they from theirs, and so on. These patterns are likely to repeat until the family becomes conscious of them and is then able to make a choice.

Although our experience of being parented in a certain way may lead to a radical difference in how we ourselves parent, the change is still generated from that experience and can still be perceived as 'ancestral'.

Like us, our parents are influenced by their own diverse experiences (including religion and culture) and, whether we share these with them or not, they will take up some space in our world.

Children also learn about themselves by *identifying* with a certain physical or behavioural trait that has been highlighted within them. For example, a child with red hair may have been observed in a temper and had that temper attributed to their hair colouring. An adult may comment that a child is just like another family member. In each case, the child may identify with that statement and, if it serves them, the behaviour may become exaggerated and adopted into the *personality*.

The position into which we are born in the family will also have a bearing on core beliefs, behaviour and subsequent *personality*. Being cast in the role of 'only child' will be a very different experience from growing up with many siblings. An older sibling might identify with being labelled as 'sensible' and 'responsible'. They might even be perceived as bossy. The youngest sibling might be forever seen as the baby and given less responsibility. If these roles suit a child, they will adopt them. If not, they will carve out new roles, but they will not be unaffected.

When there is more than one child in a household, it is common for adults to discuss and compare their perceived personalities. Parents and carers often observe and remark on behaviour, aptitude and preferences. If a child is seen to have a particular interest or talent, he or she might be encouraged to pursue this by the purchase of books or equipment. Adults do this to understand and support the children in their care. They may, of course, discourage some traits according to their own needs. This kind of behaviour influences the core beliefs of the child. The result may be either positive or negative.

A child who has experienced a sibling with a particular skill might switch that skill off in themselves and direct their attention towards something else. This is how, as children, we come to identify as 'the clever one', 'the pretty one', 'the sensible one', 'the clumsy one', 'the sporty one', 'the animal lover', 'the dancer', etc.

The way that the adults who are close to us in childhood directly interact with us can have a profound effect on core beliefs. Most of us can remember some negative words that adults used to describe us while we were growing up. We remember the ones that hurt. We also remember the ones profound enough to shape us. It is worth noting that the adults in our childhood had their own challenges to deal with, and what is important here is *our* processing of those comments and not why they were made. We will discuss the power of words in much more detail in Chapter 9.

Again, these labels are not *who we are*, but we may have identified with them and adopted them as part of our adult personality. We can also reject them and go completely the other way. They have, however, still influenced us.

If we learn to recognize where we were influenced, we are activating our *internal locus of control* (Chapter 1). *We* are then afforded the power to *choose* whether to repeat our usual patterns of behaviour to effect the same old outcome, or to *evolve!* We evolve when we take responsibility and reframe our processes. The reason why we choose to repeat our behaviours is because evolving is not our normal pattern. It feels uncomfortable. It is hard work. We will discuss this further in Chapters 8, 9 and 15 in our Core Skills section.

We have explored how the actions of those who care for us in early life can affect us. However, it is very important that we do not generalize when applying these concepts. The experience of childhood varies greatly from person to person, as does the genetic blueprint of each child processing the information. It is, therefore, difficult to predict how a child in certain circumstances will present as an adult. A child who has grown up in care and is undergoing a lot of change might experience more difficulty in forming close personal relationships than a child who has grown up with the stability of a loving home. It is also understandable that some children who are abused may enter into abusive relationships themselves. It may be that they have not learned how a loving relationship feels and do not have those skills. However, many children who have suffered difficulties go on to love furiously, appreciating bonds that were denied to them at that crucial time.

The purpose of this book is not to encourage limitation with labels or judgement. It is to inspire you to develop a good understanding as to how your personal experience of parenting may have affected you. Proceed with kindness, and know that your parents did the best that they could within their own model of the world.

Life experiences and lessons

As children, we begin by gathering information from those who are close to us within the family or childhood home. We continue to build on that data by learning from others and processing the consequences of our experiences.

When something new, unexpected or frightening happens, children react in two ways:

- **They unconsciously look to adults for the appropriate responses** – children know that adults have much more survival experience than they do and, therefore, copying adult responses is a safe bet. This can become a problem, however, if the adult in question has an irrational behavioural response to a particular stimulus (e.g. a fear of spiders); the child may well inherit that fear.
- **They select an automatic or physiological response such as blushing, running away, screaming or becoming anxious or aggressive.** As the situation plays out, if no harm comes to the child, that behaviour is unconsciously 'programmed' as the appropriate response for such a situation. For example, if you were put on the spot by a teacher at school, by being asked a question to which you did not know the answer, you may have turned red in the face. When the situation subsided, and you observed that you did not die or lose any of your limbs, you might have programmed that as your response for further situations of embarrassment. This is effective in learning how to respond, but, as we become adults, those responses can become outmoded and in need of reframing. As adults, we do not wish to blush every time we are put under pressure. We can modify our responses ourselves as we continue to learn, but sometimes our attachment to those responses is strengthened by fear and we may need help.

Children learn through experiencing the consequences of their choices. They modify and process the appropriate behaviours for survival. When something that they perceive as bad happens, they learn to avoid any behaviour that they judge to have caused it. When something good happens, such as attention from an adult, they will adopt behaviour which they deem to have led to it, in order for it to continue.

These patterns are carried into adulthood, and they are deep rooted and difficult to see, especially if we attribute them to our *personality.*

Another factor affecting our experience is the *over-culture.* This term was first coined by Dr Clarissa Pinkola Estes[2] and can be defined as the sum of the dominant cultures within society whose traditions and customs are usually followed by individuals in public. During our continuous development, we are exposed to a profusion of ideas, judgements, ideals and opinions from a diverse range of sources such as religion, media, society, social media and our peers. To preserve our safety, the usual behaviour is to go with the flow or follow the trend, unless we are trying to define ourselves as 'different'. Either way, what we are bombarded with ultimately shapes us.

When we are young, we are hard-wired to survive. Every experience that we have is logged and the outcome processed so that we can utilize the information to armour us for life.

Genetic make-up

Much of our behaviour is learned as described above. However, there is evidence that some of our behaviour is genetically inherited.[3] This suggests that we are all born with a genetic, psychological blueprint which becomes moulded by experience.

As described above, two people might have exactly the same upbringing and very similar experiences and yet process those experiences and subsequently behave very differently. They will certainly present with different personalities.

Our genetic make-up may be responsible for some of our likes and dislikes. It might also give us certain hereditary talents. We might, for example, be born with an aptitude for music or sport. What develops in the personality will depend on how we respond to our environment. If we are not given an instrument to play or sporting equipment, we may never realize that potential. The same might happen if that skill is not valued by the adults around us. The characteristics we are born with may be 'switched off' or exaggerated depending on how we are received in the outside world.

In therapy for recovering from trauma, the main emphasis is not given to the actual event, but to the *processing* of it. We may well inherit those processes genetically. We can certainly work with our processes therapeutically.

The lens through which we view the world is determined by our processing of life experiences and our genetic make-up. We often find ourselves in conflict with others. This is because our truth – that is, our model of the world – is, understandably, very different from theirs. We can experience life only through our own lens but, when we become familiar with it, we can effect change.

The purpose of this book is to encourage you to develop the high level of self-awareness required for resilience. This involves shifting your locus of control to the internal end of the spectrum. It is all about accepting responsibility for your own processes so that they can be modified to serve you. This will allow you to reach your highest potential.

In the next chapter, we will further enhance your understanding of emotions to improve your self-awareness.

3

Understanding our emotions

I don't want to be at the mercy of my emotions. I want to use them; to enjoy them, and to dominate them.

Oscar Wilde

In this chapter, we will discuss positive and negative emotions and how they are formed. We will explore the body chemistry that is associated with these emotions, and how this drives further thinking, feelings and behaviours in a positive or negative way. This is known as the cognitive behavioural cycle. We will explain why we tend to think more negatively and the effect this has on our body. Lastly, we will examine how all this knowledge can be used to combat the common addiction to negative thinking.

Emotions are feelings or body experiences. They can be either positive (pleasurable) or negative (unpleasant). There has been much research into emotions, where they come from and what causes them. They are initially felt in the body. For example, anxiety is often expressed as a tight chest or churning stomach. These symptoms can, however, be caused by something physical (e.g. asthma or a food intolerance). The difficulty lies in determining one from the other. Often, children will complain of a tummy ache when they feel anxious. These can quickly become linked for them.

The origin of thoughts

Lisa Feldman Barrett,[1] a neuroscientist, teaches that emotions do not just happen *to* us, they are actually made *by* us. Our brains use past experiences to construct our world, and emotions are a large part of our experience. This is why two people can be in the same situation but have very different reactions or emotions as a consequence of the same circumstances.[2] The emotions we feel have not been thrust upon us by external events; we have created them. Our emotions are built by our brain as we need them, and they are specific to our current thought processes. For example, people often say 'I have anxiety' whereas, in fact, thinking about anxiety triggers the release of chemicals in their body that drives the anxious feeling.

In Chapter 2, we discussed conditioning and how our core beliefs are formed. These core beliefs influence our attitudes and behaviours, they dictate how we judge ourselves and others, and they are the filter through which we view the world. According to Dr Feldman Barrett, then, core beliefs are the elements which our brain uses to construct thoughts and, ultimately, our world. Emotions are the consequence of this. Our core beliefs are deep-seated, unconscious and consistent. We believe them to be true and so it is not in our nature to question them. When we encounter a stimulus (either positive or negative), we unconsciously check it against our core beliefs and our brain responds accordingly. People with negative core beliefs are more likely to respond with negative thoughts, and those with positive core beliefs are more likely to experience positive thoughts.

Every time we experience a thought the nerve cells (also known as neurons) in our brains fire and make connections. If we repeat the thought, more and more connections are made until you have a neural network. These neural networks are continually responding to information from our body and the environment. The firing of neurons in our neural networks release chemicals (known as neurotransmitters). These then stimulate a chemical response within the body. This creates the feelings associated with emotions and prompts physiological and physical changes to prepare us for certain behaviours.

The fight/flight response is an excellent example of a cognitive behavioural cycle that is associated with anxiety. It is mediated by the autonomic nervous system which governs the body processes that we do not consciously control. It consists of two pathways, the sympathetic and the parasympathetic nervous systems, which continually respond to signals from the brain. We recognize environmental threats or stressors, we think 'danger' and our brain responds. It activates the sympathetic nervous system, stimulating the release of the fight/flight chemicals adrenaline and cortisol. Adrenaline raises our blood pressure, heart rate and respiratory rate; it dilates our pupils to maximize our vision and prepares our muscles for movement. We become breathless and sweaty; we feel our heart racing and our muscles trembling. We are primed and ready for action. If we needed to run away or fight, these physiological changes would be very useful; otherwise they merely serve to make us feel uncomfortable and even unwell. Cortisol down-regulates the systems we do not need in fight/flight, such as our digestion, the immune system and reproduction. When the threat has gone, activation of the parasympathetic nervous system down-regulates the stress hormones, the physical symptoms settle, and our body processes return to normal function. This is known as the relaxation response.[3] The fight/flight response is a perfect cycle of thoughts (perception of danger), feelings (fight/flight chemical effects) and behaviours (physical changes in response to the chemicals).

Positive stimuli and thoughts activate neurons that stimulate the release of different neurotransmitters: serotonin and dopamine. Serotonin has effects on many body systems. It regulates mood and makes us feel happier; it affects memory, sexual desire and function; it helps us sleep and aids digestion, reducing our appetite as we eat.

Dopamine is released during pleasurable activities such as eating and sex. It is part of the brain's motivation and reward system. It is important for smooth coordinated movement, memory, attention, focus and problem solving. Low levels of dopamine are associated with pain.

The neurotransmitters released by our thoughts also affect other parts of the brain. Our prefrontal cortex is like a control centre. It collects information from other areas of the brain and interprets this. It is important in our decision making and impulse control. It works to coordinate behaviour (e.g. 'I need to move the top two parcels to get to the bottom one'). It also allows us to consider the ramifications of our actions (e.g. 'If I pull the bottom parcel out the others will fall on me!'). Brain imaging experiments in neuroplasticity show that negative thoughts reduce activity in the prefrontal cortex, limiting our ability to think and control the autonomic nervous system responses. Positive thoughts are associated with increased activity in this region, improving our decision making.

In life, the things we give attention to get bigger, and this is true even in neural activity. The more negative thoughts we have, the more stress chemicals are released, and the less our prefrontal cortex can control that release. This results in more negative feelings and physical symptoms, which, in turn, drives negative behaviours such as avoidance, impulsivity and poor decision making. The negative feelings and behaviours feed back into our thoughts, and the cycle goes round and round in a negative spiral. Positive thoughts stimulate the release of feel-good chemicals and our prefrontal cortex is stimulated; we have pleasurable feelings, we feel happier, and our behaviours respond with open, considered actions that make us and others think and feel good, and so the positive spiral is formed. This cognitive behavioural model explains the complex relationship between our core beliefs and our thoughts, feelings and behaviours.

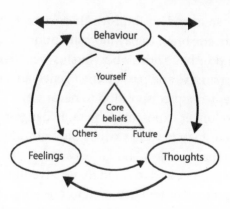

Why we think negatively

Let us now examine why it appears to be human nature to think in a negative way. Our brains are predisposed to respond to negative stimuli above positive. This concept forms part of a recognized psychological phenomenon known as the *negativity bias*. This was first discussed in the 1970s by Kanouse et al.,[4] and, since then, years of research has shown multiple examples. Negative traits in a person have more of an impression on those judging them. Voting behaviour has been shown to be more influenced by negative information than positive – meaning a scandal about one candidate is more likely to affect our decision than a positive story about another. Loss aversion experiments conclude that we are more upset by losing money than we are by winning the same amount. When remembering events, people are more likely to remember negative experiences than positive.[5] Negative news videos produce a bigger reaction from the audience than positive. We attend to, use and learn from negative stimuli more than positive ones (e.g. from punishment more than praise!). Observational studies of children have also shown that children learn this negativity bias as they develop.

Thousands of years ago, our ancestors lived in a very dangerous world. They had to be alert at all times to potential threats.

For safety reasons and to improve their chances of survival, it made sense for the brain to pay more attention to negative information than positive. Those whose brains were best at this were more likely to survive and pass on their genes, and, consequently, we have inherited a predisposition to negativity.

We are no longer exposed to the same dangers as prehistoric humans. There may be times when the fight/flight response is required, but these are few and far between. So, we have a brain predisposed to notice and respond to negative stimuli, and a very fast threat response system designed to prepare us for action.

What does this mean for us? Well, we have all experienced our fight/flight system in action; we feel the symptoms described above when we stand at the front and speak, attend a job interview or get involved in conflict. When we think negatively about a situation, we are effectively labelling it as a threat. Our autonomic nervous system does not know the difference between a clear and present danger and performance anxiety. If we perceive everyday events as threats, then our brain will keep responding accordingly. We can end up almost permanently in fight/flight mode with high levels of stress hormones relentlessly circulating in our bodies. This has significant consequences. Persistently high levels of cortisol and adrenaline contribute to digestive problems, headaches, sleep disturbances, cognitive impairment and weight gain. They also increase the risk of developing cardiovascular disease, anxiety and depression.

Our threat response can become so heightened that a danger does not even need to occur to trigger the stress hormone release! Negative thoughts in the form of memories of something that happened in the past, or imaginings of something that might happen in the future, will set it off. Remembered and imagined events produce the same threat response as the event itself. Reliving a trauma or remembering a mistake makes us feel the same sick gut feeling and sets our heart racing. Imagining or rehearsing a difficult interaction or feeling a body lump and imagining the worst does the same. Chemically, our perception becomes our reality.

In addition to this, if the core beliefs that lie at the heart of our perception are negative, then we will continually look for evidence that proves they are true, even to the point of ignoring any evidence to the contrary. For example, a common negative core belief is that of being unworthy. People who have this core belief will focus their *attention* on anything that suggests they are not good enough. An unsuccessful job interview will clearly reinforce this core belief, but it can, and often does, get more extreme. We may start to perceive all feedback as negative, and we can even come to interpret an expression on another person's face as being about us. The expression is much more likely to be about something else entirely, but we distort the evidence to reinforce our belief.

It is important to note here that memory cannot always be relied upon as truth, especially where emotions are involved. We can remember past events with 'rose-coloured glasses' when we want to complain about the present. Similarly, we can distort a memory of our past action, again to punish ourselves and reinforce negative core beliefs.

Eckhart Tolle describes a phenomenon that he calls 'the pain body'.[6] This is an accumulation of all the negative things that have happened in our lives that are unresolved. Our pain body, then, is the filter through which we view the world, and this will, of course, affect our thoughts, making them more negative. Tolle also states that our pain body makes us crave negativity, driving our thoughts, feelings and behaviours into the negative spiral. This may be because we are searching for resolution or, again, because we are seeking to confirm negative core beliefs. This is what drives the habitual repetition and revisiting of negative situations. We experience pain body when we recruit others to our cause and have our 'right' to feel hurt validated.

In fact, we can become so used to the high levels of adrenaline circulating in our body that we become addicted to them. We are all adrenaline junkies. Some of us get our high from extreme sports, some of us from extreme negative thinking. The sporting activities bring with them the balancing effect of serotonin and dopamine; the negative thinking does not.

In conclusion, we are predisposed to think negatively due to evolution. Our core beliefs developed in childhood can be negative, and we continually look for evidence that reinforces those beliefs. We become addicted to our negative body chemistry and so choose to think more negatively in order to stimulate the release of more of those chemicals. These thoughts and feelings repeated over and over again generate negative patterns of behaviour. The behaviours and feelings drive more negative thoughts, and our cognitive behavioural cycles become habitual. They then dictate what we draw towards us and what becomes manifest in our lives. We will explore the Universal Law of Manifestation in the next chapter.

Positive thoughts

Let us now explore the effect of positive cognitive behavioural cycles. Barbara Fredrickson studies positivity. She has proven that positive emotions promote creativity and openness and foster positive relationships. She has shown that being positive opens our mind to new possibilities and this allows us to learn new skills and forge new relationships; this is her 'broaden and build' model.[7] Positive emotions improve performance on tests and in our cognition. Increasing positive thoughts allows us to be more mindful.

Positive thoughts are the key to breaking the negative spiral we often indulge in. The best place to start generating positive thoughts is to be *grateful for what you already have*. Starting here means that you do not need to *acquire* or *change* anything.

Gratitude is recognized across cultures. In shamanic practice it is seen as one of the gifts we are born with. Every time we are grateful, we are open to receiving abundance from the universe.

Robert Emmons, a professor of psychology at the University of California, Davis, has been studying gratitude for many years in thousands of test subjects. MRI scans of the brain when people are feeling grateful shows activity in multiple areas, including the reward centre and the hypothalamus. The hypothalamus secretes dopamine, which we know is a 'feel good' neurotransmitter. Emmons's research has demonstrated physical, psychological and social benefits to gratitude,[8] including a significant reduction in depression, feelings of hopelessness in suicidal patients and circulating levels of cortisol. He also noted a 25 per cent reduction in fat intake in study subjects, and a 10 per cent improvement in the quality of sleep in patients suffering from chronic pain.

Grateful people have a stronger immune system, they have a better tolerance to pain, they eat better and are more likely to exercise. They are more positive and more alert, they are more optimistic and more likely to experiences feelings of joy and pleasure. Grateful people are more generous and compassionate, more forgiving and less likely to feel lonely. In Part 3 there are tools to help you start to cultivate gratitude and, with it, resilience.

In conclusion, understanding the complex relationship between thoughts, feelings and behaviours gives us an opportunity to intervene. Dr Feldman-Barrett admits the implications of her research are uncomfortable: to accept that we are ultimately responsible for how we feel is hard to hear, but with great *responsibility* comes great *power*. If we ultimately create our emotions, then we have control over how we feel: we can therefore consciously choose to feel better! From her research, to affect our emotions we need to make sure our brain has positive information to work with. We are not advocating ignoring our negative thoughts; in fact, this has been proven to be detrimental.[9] What we are saying is that we must be conscious of our thoughts as much as possible. As Dr Feldman-Barrett says, 'We are the architects of our own experience.'

Being grateful is an easy way to generate positive thoughts. Being aware of our core beliefs and understanding how they are influencing our thoughts empowers us to take those core beliefs and reframe them positively. Recognizing negative thoughts and questioning them allows us to discount them. Analysing our fears and truly examining the evidence for and against them helps us reframe them. Staying in the present moment helps us to observe our thoughts without reacting to them, while experiments have shown that mindfulness increases connectivity in our prefrontal cortex, decreasing our impulsivity and improving our decision making.

Part 2 covers the essential core skills required to question and reframe core beliefs and practise mindfulness. Part 3 is rich with practical tools to help you be more present, be more grateful, and become aware of and reframe your thoughts, feelings and behaviours – allowing you to access the power of positivity.

In the next chapter, we will delve even more deeply into self-awareness by exploring the universal laws.

4

Introducing the universal laws

The universe is always listening ... feel it, get consumed with
its generosity and power ... good things are coming!

Wesam Fawzi

A universal law is something which applies to us, whether we
believe in its existence or not. There is much varied and fascinating literature detailing and categorizing a generous number
of universal spiritual laws.

Publications about spiritual laws are numerous and diverse.
They are usually comprised of a set of rules, varying in number
and description, which have been identified and explored by
authors with an interest in the human psyche and its interactions
within the universe. They all operate on the principle of 'cause and
effect'. They are often seen as the naturally existing mechanisms
which bring the universe back into balance. There is no doubt
that, however these laws are perceived and understood, they are all
connected and constantly at play throughout our lives.

For the purpose of this book, we have chosen to focus on
the key concepts that are most relevant to cultivating resilience
in everyday life. We will explore the universal laws of *reflection*,
attraction, *intention*, *attention*, *detachment* and *manifestation*.

The Universal Law of Reflection

The Universal Law of Reflection states: 'Everything in the universe
that enters my awareness is a reflection of part of my Self.'

The universe contains everything in existence. There is
infinitely more information than can be processed by the

human mind. We cannot, at any time, perceive everything. What then leads us to *choose* what we see? Why do we notice certain things and not others?

We see the aspects of the universe that reflect all parts of the Self.

The universe behaves like a mirror. When we like and approve of someone, we are appreciating in them qualities that we appreciate in ourselves. Conversely, when someone shows qualities that we dislike or that make us uncomfortable, we are seeing parts of the Self that we dislike, and we are unpleasantly provoked.

When we have gone to such great lengths to hide and deny those parts that they are no longer evident in our *personality*, they reside in our *shadow*. We will explore this concept in greater depth in Chapter 5.

The Universal Law of Reflection teaches that *when someone bothers you, it is your problem.* It is highlighting where you need to work on yourself. If you acknowledge and accept those parts of the Self that feel uncomfortable when reflected, the irritation with the other person will dissolve.

Taking responsibility for our responses and reactions is the ultimate shift of our *locus of control* towards the internal end of the spectrum. When we are responsible, we retain our power. No one and nothing external can affect our emotions. This is true resilience.

When we are responsible, we can undertake to do the work.

When something enters our consciousness, it is signposting us towards something within ourselves.

The Universal Law of Attraction (*like attracts like*)

The Universal Law of Attraction is the concept of matching the energy/vibration of our thoughts with that which we wish to draw towards us in life.

This teaching suggests that the direction in which we focus our thoughts dictates what comes into our lives. It suggests that positive thinking attracts positive experiences and that negative thinking attracts negative ones. Most of us can identify with experiences in our lives where we have dreaded the worst scenario, only to find it hurtling towards us at great speed despite it being the least likely outcome.

According to the Universal Law of Attraction, fear attracts fear and love attracts love. Need attracts need and abundance attracts abundance, and so on. It encourages us to watch our *thoughts*. Remember that thoughts arise from *core beliefs*.

- People who *believe* that they are capable of great things usually go on to achieve them.
- People who *believe* that they have no luck often suffer misfortune.
- People who *believe* that they are not deserving of wealth rarely experience abundance.

John has had the unfortunate experience of being made redundant. He is in desperate need of another job. His family's survival depends on it. There are no other options for feeding and housing them. In this situation, there is a great deal at stake for him and his thoughts of what will happen if he fails reinforce fearful and negative emotions within him. Remember that, in the cognitive behavioural cycle, *thoughts lead to emotions which in turn lead to behaviours*. Here his behaviour will be, understandably, negatively affected by the amount of need. Need has its roots in fear.

It has been shown that an astounding 93 per cent of communication is non-verbal.[1] It would, therefore, be exceedingly difficult for John to present himself at interview in the most positive and confident light. He is projecting *need*. John's competitor, however, is in more affluent circumstances, with plenty of wealth to fall back on should he fail. He has experienced a successful career and perceives himself to be a great asset to any organization. He is projecting *wealth* and *success*. He believes that he is both talented and blessed, and is far more likely to present as a confident and accomplished candidate.

To activate the Universal Law of Attraction in a positive way, we must reframe our negative beliefs and align our emotions with those that we wish to feel at the outcome. Simply altering our behaviour to get what we want, while harbouring our old negative core beliefs, will not result in success. We cannot cheat the universe.

If we want something, *we must live as if we already have it*, and it will be ours.

If we want to be satisfied with our lives, then *we must be grateful for what we already have*.

The Universal Law of Manifestation

A clearly visualized and stated intention, given appropriate attention followed by emotional detachment, will become manifest.

Look around at your possessions. Everything that you see began as a conscious thought in a human mind. How, then, were the wheels set in motion for it to become a physical manifestation?

They activated this law.

To activate the Universal Law of Manifestation, we must set a clear, pure *intention*, give it our full *attention*, and emotionally *detach* from the outcome. These individual laws are explained in more depth below.

The Universal Law of Intention (I focus my thoughts on exactly what I want)

Intention *is the first requirement for* **manifestation**. *We have heard it said that intention is everything.*

Consider an arrowhead as pure potential. It holds all the possibilities. At its point is the moment of *manifestation*. The moment that the archer releases the potential, her attention is brought entirely to the point of the arrow and its target – just like an acupuncturist's focus is entirely on the point of the needle and the area intended for healing.

But before that moment, the archer must have intention. Without intention, the arrow has no direction and all the energy in firing it will be absorbed somewhere in its aimless journey. What manifests has no precision. It may cause harm. It may pass unnoticed.

Before taking action, we must clearly set our *intention*. It must be worded thoughtfully using simple, precise language. We must be very honest about what it is that we *really* want. This will improve the chances of our project coming to fruition. It will also ensure that the results will be exact.

We may wish to set a time limit by which we hope to see results. It is important to remember to allow for external limitations over which we have no control. We can then ask, 'Is this precisely what I want to happen?'

When we put our energy into a project with no clear intention, we manifest *chaos*.

We must be mindful of making clear, pure *intentions*.

The Universal Law of Attention (whatever I give attention to in my life gets bigger)

Attention is the second requirement for **manifestation.** *Whatever we choose to focus more of our attention on takes up a proportionately larger space in our consciousness.*

This law can be applied in a negative way, as we see in the following case study:

Anne has recently moved into a beautiful new house. She likes her neighbours. She has settled in well, and she can see herself being happy there for many years to come. Everything is rosy. Anne's friend then comes to visit. As she proudly shows him around her cosy new home, he asks her whether she is irritated by the sound of music and chatter coming through the wall from the next-door house. She had not been aware of the noise until it was mentioned. After his visit, she begins to worry that the neighbours will not be kind enough to turn their music down at night and moderate their socializing. In the weeks that follow, these fears take up a large proportion of her conscious thinking. As a consequence, the music appears to her to get louder and more invasive. Her neighbours seem to be socializing all the time.

Negative thoughts lead to negative emotions, which, in turn, lead to negative behaviours. Before she knows it, her life appears to be consumed by this terrible issue. She confronts her neighbours, who do not react well as they perceive that their behaviour is reasonable. When Anne moved in, she perceived it that way, too. She allowed her friend's comments to provoke a reframing of her thoughts from positive to negative. This was driven by the fear that everything was not as perfect as she had originally perceived. That fear then drove her to further negative thinking. It also caused her to give much of her attention to the problem, which took up more and more space in her psyche until she was consumed by it.

To explore the positive application of the Universal Law of Attention, let us once again discuss our archer. Once the archer knows his target, he can fire his arrow. He cannot, however, do this effectively without a good bow.

He must put his **attention** towards the quality and maintenance of his equipment. He must make sure, not just that it is fit for purpose, but that it is superbly crafted from the best materials and supremely designed.

This will help to ensure the success of his quest. He must tune the bow, wax the string, and check the riser. This is *attention*. It ensures *manifestation* of *intention*. The more *attention* he gives, the more finely tuned and exquisite his bow and arrow become; the more positive his thinking; the stronger his faith in them; the better his aim. The more assured his success.

Universal laws are so named because they apply across the board. When we are in love, we may give it our full attention and be consumed by it. The same applies with pain.

We must *consciously choose* where we put our *attention*.

The more *attention* we give to something, the more space it will take up in our lives and the larger it will become.

The Universal Law of Detachment (detachment is a prerequisite to enlightenment)[2]

*Detachment is the third and final requirement for **manifestation**. When we emotionally detach from an outcome, we release it to become subject to universal law.*

When we are emotionally bound to something or someone, we make them responsible for how we feel. This includes any outcome of a situation in which we have invested our time, energy and *attention*. It is understandable that we would emotionally invest in a situation for which we have taken the trouble to set a clear, pure *intention* and focused a large amount of *attention*. However, we *must* complete the process by remembering to emotionally *detach*. By remaining attached we hold on to it with hope and fear, thereby obstructing the process. We revisit it. A farmer does not dig up her seeds after planting to check that they are germinating in the hope that they are, and in fear that they are not. She pays *attention* to them – giving them water and warmth and protecting them from predators. Still, she visualizes how healthy and sturdy they will be on the day that they reach their full height.

When we are *attached* to an outcome, it has power over us. We are bound to it and blocked from moving forward.

By detaching, we move our *locus of control* from the external to internal end of our spectrum, thereby improving our chances of becoming more resilient.

Throughout life we can observe our own attachments. We can consciously choose when to remain attached and when to *detach*, for the greater good of all.

When we wish our projects to become manifest, we must remember to emotionally *detach* from the outcome and send it out to the universe.

The Universal Law of Manifestation (intention + attention + detachment = manifestation)

For an intention to become manifest, we must hold a clear vision of the desired outcome while remaining emotionally detached from it. We need to *know* that the outcome is assured.

Amanda works part-time as a teacher. She has concerns about the environment and the quality of the food that she buys from the supermarket. She worries about pesticides. She usually buys organic produce but this has become expensive. She wonders whether she could grow her own vegetables.

She has an ornamental garden which will not easily convert into a vegetable patch; she has limited time during the week due to her work and social commitments; she has very little horticultural knowledge and is not sure how to begin.

Without intention, Amanda is unlikely to take action. She already has a busy schedule and little knowledge about the subject. Although she would like to grow food, her resistance to change is high. This leads to her becoming discouraged and putting it off until another time. Another time is unlikely to present itself, since she has no plans to change her current situation.

After months of toying with the idea, Amanda decides that growing her own food really is a priority for her. She feels motivated. She asks herself, 'What is my intention? I intend to have begun growing my own vegetables within the next 12 months.'

She does not specify where or how so that she is not limited by her own circumstances. She does, however, give herself the time limit of a full year to allow for seasonal variety and so that its manifestation is no longer postponed. She has thoughtfully worded her intention.

She visualizes a manageable patch of earth crammed full of luscious greens, reds, oranges and yellows. It is done! Now she must address the attention she needs to give to the situation, in order for her intention to become manifest.

She asks herself, 'What do I need to give my attention to? I need to convert my garden or find an area of land for rent on which to grow vegetables. I need to acquire the horticultural knowledge to begin cultivating soil and growing plants. I need to purchase or borrow appropriate equipment. I need to buy seeds and/or plants.

I need to find time in my busy week to water, feed and, eventually, harvest my produce.'

She begins to take action. After deciding that she enjoys sitting in her ornamental garden on warm weekend afternoons, she decides to enquire at the local parish council about the possibility of renting one of the allotments, which are a short walk away from her house. She puts her name on the list and is soon able to take on a small plot to suit her needs. She imagines the plot teeming with nutritious produce.

She researches allotment keeping on the Internet. She examines her weekly schedule and makes small adjustments in order to free up time for gardening. Surprisingly, this does not involve much sacrificing of other activities as she is able to pick out slots in her week where her time was not being used effectively. She joins the local gardening club in the village hall, where she makes new friends who delight in sharing with her their secrets and tips on the growing of tasty, healthy vegetables. Some of her friends use the same allotments as she does and offer to lend her their gardening equipment so that she can invest in her own over time. She is given seeds and cuttings by her new friends. She also enjoys shopping around in the local garden centres for new and exciting varieties.

Amanda plants her seeds and cuttings; she tends to them, knowing that they will grow. She does not worry about the success of her project. Amanda begins to see results quickly, and within the year she has become a member of the gardening community and successfully grown many varieties of vegetables.

In conclusion, human existence is bound by universal law. It is by *observing* our own part in the universe and consciously *choosing* our responses that we cultivate self-awareness, leading to resilience and improved wellbeing.

When we activate the universal laws, the universe shifts accordingly. We should aim to activate them consciously for the greater good.

In the next chapter, as promised, we will explain how you can honour your shadow.

5

Honouring your shadow

One does not become enlightened by imagining figures of light, but by making the darkness conscious.

Carl Jung

When we are born we are *whole*, with equal amounts of all things and with no characteristic that can be deemed either good or bad. As infants, however, we are hard-wired to survive. This means that we must seek the *approval* of those caring for us and avoid rejection at all costs. Rejection to a helpless child means *death*, and so *acceptance* equals *survival*. As we develop, we respond to the behaviour and reactions of those around us. We learn to *embody* the behaviours and characteristics that gain positive reactions and approval, and *disown* and *put away* those parts of us which do not. We *choose* which aspects of the Self we will accept and develop as *personality*, and the parts that are rejected collectively become our *shadow*. When they are not acknowledged or addressed, they can rise to the surface and create obstacles in our daily lives.

The concept of the shadow has been around for hundreds of years. You will find reference to it in the work of the thirteenth century Persian poet Rumi[1] and it has been expanded upon as a valuable therapeutic tool by the likes of both Jung and Freud.

Why, then, does it seem to be less well known than other phenomena of the psyche?

Honouring our shadow is one of the most valuable practices in the quest for personal enlightenment. However, so-called 'shadow work' can be uncomfortable, which may explain why so few people have heard of it. We believe this to be unfortunate because it offers profound personal insight and *exceptional* growth.

As we discussed in Chapter 2, early in our childhood we begin to process the reactions and responses to our behaviour of the influential people in our lives. We learn to discern between approval and disapproval. We then put away aspects of ourselves that do not fit what we have perceived to be the 'accepted' model. These are aspects of the Self revealed in behaviour which has invoked displeasure, irritation or even anger in others and, subsequently, shame within us. This process greatly influences the development of our *personality* and how we present to the outside world. To avoid rejection, we present a 'sanitized' version of the unabridged Self. For at least the early part of our lives, that version of the Self is *who we believe that we are*. It sits comfortably within our understanding of the way that things *should* be and our unique model of the world. Most importantly, we feel *safe* when we exist within these parameters. The illusion of safety, however, is quickly challenged when we are confronted with a true reflection of certain parts of the Self.

To create a version of the Self that we believe to be 'acceptable' to the world, we must disown the parts of ourselves that do not appear to fit. We reject the whole, unabridged Self with all its potential, in favour of developing a personality comprising a collection of 'approved' behaviours and characteristics. Those rejected parts of the Self remain but are disowned by us and become our shadow.

We measure our self-worth by how successful we are in creating the 'acceptable' Self (by adapting to the responses of those key figures in our early external environment). Our core beliefs about the Self are also rooted here.

How, then, do we recognize our shadow?

This phenomenon is easier to see in others than in one's own Self because there is little emotional cost to observing the processes of those around us. When we dare to look at our own processes, there is much at stake. We have spent a lifetime building and embodying the person *we think we are* to ensure survival and, later, success. When we acknowledge the shadow, we are pulling at the foundations of everything that we have encouraged ourselves and others to believe.

When we are introduced to someone and are asked to describe ourselves, we will strongly focus on those characteristics that we are comfortable with. We will illustrate the approved version of ourselves and often, unconsciously, go to great lengths to hide or deny our shadow. Most of us are aware of the existence of the shadow parts of ourselves only when we are confronted with a reflection of them in someone else.

People will reveal to you everything about their light and shadow parts when they are asked to describe their own personality. They do this by telling you what they are and what they are not. They are unconsciously painting a picture of how they perceive themselves and would like to be perceived; this includes what they do not want to acknowledge. This is affirmation. They are also managing your expectations so that their shadow is not revealed.

For example, someone who firmly insists that they are not an extrovert may have been shown displeasure in response to their gregarious behaviour when young. Perhaps they were told that children should be seen and not heard, and therefore pushed their extrovert Self firmly away. By telling you what they are not, they may well be adjusting your expectations of them so that you do not suggest anything that may pull back the veil.

Someone who tells you that they are not judgemental is putting their hand over the judge in their shadow. If we dislike the mean-spirited habits of a family member, we are confronted with the part of us that is capable of being mean.

When we teach this concept in workshops, we are often challenged. The most difficult example we have been faced with is that of abuse. People ask, 'If I am appalled by the thoughts of child abuse, does that mean that a part of me is an abuser?'

We answer by explaining that when we are uncomfortably provoked by the behaviour of someone else, we are seeing our own shadow reflected. The more uncomfortable we are, the deeper we have buried that part of the Self. Witnessing the characteristics required for that behaviour in others reminds us that they are still there within us. We draw back in revulsion when we witness cruelty, abuse, theft and violence in their worst forms. However, in the right circumstances, *we are all capable of the cruelty, manipulation and selfishness that this sort of behaviour requires.*

When we witness such behaviour, we feel repulsed because it reflects our shadow. However, when we engage our powers of observation, we can learn to recognize when this has happened and *sit with it.* Observing the shadow is the first step. This is often enough to affect positive change. When we acknowledge our shadow, the discomfort is reduced. We can take this further by asking ourselves a question like 'What are the characteristics demonstrated in this behaviour?' We can then follow up with: 'Where in my life do I show these characteristics?' When we have identified those parts of the shadow Self, we can learn to *accept* them. By doing this we are honouring the *whole* Self rather than only the parts that are in the *light.*

When we honour the whole Self, we are no longer provoked by the behaviour of others. This is because we are no longer judging ourselves or them, and so, in turn, their behaviour does not trigger us. When we are unaffected by the behaviour of others, we are resilient.

Shadow work is challenging, raw and often uncomfortable, but the results can be ground-breaking. It can liberate us from past limitations and labels that we have imposed on ourselves in the search for approval. We can therefore move forward into *self-acceptance.*

A move from requiring *external acceptance* to *self-acceptance* will shift the *locus of control* towards the internal end of the spectrum. As we discussed in Chapter 1, developing self-awareness and fostering a strong internal locus of control is essential to improving our resilience.

Understanding that someone's behaviour uncomfortably provoking us can provide fertile ground for our growth and progress is a superpower!

In the next chapter, we will further explore the psyche by discussing it in terms of archetypes.

6

Identifying archetypes

If you know how to perceive the world in archetypes, through archetypes – everything changes. Everything!

Caroline Myss

In this chapter, we will discuss how fear is present in all situations but, when we are stuck, it is likely that a part of our psyche has managed to block us from moving forward. These parts of the psyche can be recognized as the four 'survival archetypes' described by Caroline Myss.

The concept of archetypes in the human psyche was first described in about 1919 by the Swiss psychologist and psychiatrist Carl Jung. Archetypes are best described as specific individual collections of characteristics, traits and behavioural patterns which are typically seen together as a group. They are used in psychoanalysis as universal symbols which help us to understand aspects of the human psyche. When we first begin to learn about them, they seem to present as caricatures of well-known personality types.

Jung believed that archetypes were innate, universal and hereditary. He rejected the idea that each human being is born a blank slate and shaped only by experience. Modern Jungian psychology continues to teach that every human psyche is comprised of a considerable number of these archetypes, and that human experience and processing will dictate which of our archetypes are evident in our personality and which ones we supress.

The concept of archetypes is widely understood and highly valued as a therapeutic framework and tool in the modern world.

Some better-known archetypes include the Mother, the Father, the Hero, the Caregiver, the Rebel, the Explorer, the

Jester, the Magician, the King, the Queen, the Knight, the Damsel, the Sorcerer, the Healer, the Princess and the Judge. When studying archetypes, we can see that there is a vast and growing list to choose from. Modern experts suggest that this list evolves alongside humanity, and new archetypes continue to be identified all the time.

The reason that descriptions of archetypes read like caricatures is that we find them in their purest form in stories. They are part of the language of human symbols, and since ancient times they have been used to convey hidden messages in both art and literature. We understand and process our lessons much more readily when we experience them by watching the latest blockbuster or find them wrapped up in an old tale that has been handed down through the generations.

In many of her publications, Dr Clarissa Pinkola Estes teaches us about the power of fairy tales as *medicine*. Across all the world's diverse cultures run common themes and archetypes within inherited storytelling. We must not forget the power of symbols in human evolution, lest we lose touch with centuries of ancestral wisdom and, indeed, our own intuition.

When we become absorbed in a story, we *identify* with its characters and whatever difficulties they find themselves in. This is because of the *Universal Law of Reflection* (see Chapter 5). Stories are rich with archetypal characters in which we can see the Self reflected. The twisting of the plot and the plight of the characters exists to teach us. This is why, at the end, we ask children, 'Now, what was the *moral* of that story? What did you *learn?*'

The vast world of archetypes is rich, fascinating and full of wisdom.

For the purpose of this book, we have chosen to focus on four archetypes, because they are recognized as the parts of the Self that stop us from moving forward. We believe acknowledging them has a profound impact on our ability to cultivate resilience in everyday life. These are the four 'survival archetypes' as first described by Caroline Myss in her publication *The Language of Archetypes*.[1] Survival archetypes are aspects of the psyche which are activated to step in to block our progress when a response of *fear* has been provoked within us.

Before we explore the four survival archetypes, let's talk about fear. Most of the suffering in the world has its roots in fear. Eckhart Tolle tells us that, 'Most fear is created through leaving the present moment mentally and projecting into the future.'[2] He explains that fear is created when our imagined future is negative. Hope is created when it is positive. The presence of hope can quickly become the fear that we will be denied that positive future.

Fear can look and feel like other emotions such as anger, jealousy, resentment or irritation. It arises at the point where we perceive that we may lose something that is important to us. These things include health, finance, identity, purpose, loved ones, success of a project and even our own precious time. This is projection. When we allow ourselves to come into the present moment, we have not lost anything at all.

As we know, when we feel fear our body chemistry changes. Levels of cortisol and adrenaline rise. Our ancestors made good use of these chemical changes, acting on the stimulus of fear, by running away or fighting whatever was threatening them. In modern society, human fear continues to exist. It is, however, stimulated by much wider, more varied sources – sources which are quite different from those of primitive humans.

We find ourselves moved into a state of fear when we listen to the news or social media, read updates on email, participate in WhatsApp groups, and so on. This is not an immediate fight/flight situation. It is projection. Here, when our fight/flight response is triggered, we do not respond in a physical way, burning off the stress hormones. This means that they are circulating in our system for longer. As we discussed in Chapter 3, this has long-term, negative consequences for us.

We should never be without fear. It keeps us safe, and our survival depends on it. We should always acknowledge it as our old friend when it reaches our awareness. Fear is present in all situations, but, as we have already discussed, when we become stuck it is likely that a part of our psyche has managed to block us from moving forward.

This type of response is evoked when our core beliefs about the Self are challenged. When this happens, we unconsciously *know that our life is going to change*. We are fearful even when the change is for the good. It is human nature to crave safety. Where we are now is *known*. Even if it is a horrible situation, it is *known*. Change is unknown and therefore could be perceived as perilous. We have no frame of reference for how to behave in a changed situation.

According to Myss, the four survival archetypes are *all* present within *all* of us.[3] As with other archetypes, some will be more evident in our personality than others. We can actually choose to activate them if we want to. Understanding and working with the survival archetypes is a skill. Again, the key is to be aware of them so you are consciously choosing whether or not to allow them to influence your thoughts, feelings and behaviours. When we are not conscious of them, we are at their mercy. They block our progress and we wonder why we are struggling to move forward.

The four survival archetypes

All archetypes have both positive and negative characteristics. We all have the power to display either. Below we have described the four survival archetypes in their most negative form to illustrate how they can place obstacles in our path.

The Child

This is a complex archetype which can be subdivided into several different categories. We invoke the child and halt our progress when we give our power to authority. We may profess not to have the knowledge or skill to handle the situation. Common characteristics include the constant need for attention and approval, craving the need for protection and nurture, resigned helplessness, powerlessness, refusal to gain knowledge or understanding of the situation, vulnerability, and refusing to act without authority or permission.

The Victim

This is where *we* block our progress by affirming that *we* cannot change anything; that nothing in the situation is within our control and that, therefore, taking action would be pointless. Common characteristics include blaming others and external circumstances, self-pity, envy, affirming powerlessness, refusal to take control, labelling ourselves and accepting labels from others, invoking pity, affirming symptoms and diagnoses, repetitive complaining, refusal to take responsibility, resigned helplessness, affirming pain and loss, and recruiting allies to validate our suffering.

The Prostitute

This archetype can be seen when moving forward is perceived to risk a loss of wealth, comfort, status or reputation. It can also be invoked when remaining stuck provides material gain. It can present as a money block – where someone will not invest materially in a project and, thereby, stop its progress. Common characteristics include selling out, staying in a situation because of a desire for financial security or material comfort, buying another person's loyalty, compromising others to gain power over them, profiting from our own or someone else's negative experience (particularly when we are in a position of power), and compromising moral values for material gain.

The Saboteur

This is where we step into a situation to spoil or ruin things for ourselves with damaging behaviour. Ultimately, it comes from the negative core belief that we are not worthy or are defective. Along with a deep-rooted belief that we will fail, there is often a compulsion to speed up the process. Common characteristics include undermining plans, refusal to do the work required, procrastination, focusing on failure, visualizing negative outcomes (activating the Universal Law of Attraction), paranoia and taking offence when none was intended, imaging negativity in others' behaviour, engaging in destructive behaviour, creating conflict and failing to speak up.

Most of us will keenly identify with at least one, or possibly two, of these archetypes for survival within our psyche. It is important to remember that when we notice them in the behaviour of others, *it is because they are reflecting those archetypes and behaviours within us*. If we are *judging* someone for their behaviour, the corresponding archetype is certainly in our shadow.

We all have the capacity to invoke any of the four survival archetypes. They serve to keep us safe by preventing us from moving forward into unknown territory. However, you will recognize that the characteristics associated with them are consistent with an external locus of control. We can internalize our locus of control by recognizing any situation where we have unconsciously obstructed our own progress because of fear. We can then acknowledge which one of our survival archetypes is coming into play. We then have the opportunity to choose whether to let it run or not.

Observing the presence of our survival archetypes where fear has been provoked is a key skill in taking control of our behaviour and responses. It is by consciously *choosing* our responses to fear that we cultivate resilience and remove obstacles to progress. We will show you how to observe and choose in Chapter 8.

What follows is the final chapter of Part 1, our theory section. We have discussed self-awareness in detail. We now focus on the balance of power within relationships.

7

The balance of power in communication

Mastering others is strength. Mastering yourself is true power.

Tao Te Ching

In this chapter, we will explore the theory of the power dynamics that exist in all our interactions.

In the 1970s, Albert Mehrabian[1] established that an astonishing 93 per cent of communication is non-verbal – 38 per cent being tone of voice and 55 per cent body language. In other words, it is not so much what you say as how you say it. It is vital to remember that *we are always expressing our intentions and desires, even when we are not speaking them.*

In Chapter 1, we described our locus of control – how much we believed we are in control of our life. An extension of this belief is our *locus of power*. When our locus of power is *internal*, we believe *we* retain control of our thoughts, feelings and behaviours. When it is *external*, we believe that *others* affect them. Our locus of power sits somewhere along the spectrum and it moves, depending on the situation.

Within all our communications there is also a *relational locus of power*, which describes where or with whom in the interaction the power resides. In this context, 'power' is the ability to affect the outcome of the interaction. This concept is also a spectrum. It lies between the two parties and the power in the interaction sits somewhere along it.

In any relationship, each party has his or her own *personal* locus of power which is, in fact, their locus of control, and within the interaction there is a further *relational* locus of power. This is the locus of power that we are referring to in this chapter. Equality within the power dynamic indicates a healthy relationship. This requires a more internal personal locus of control in both parties and a central relational locus of power.

When we approach someone to communicate with them, we are seeking either to gain information or to impart it. We are also usually seeking a *response*. Even if we are simply imparting information, we still seek a response in the form of acknowledgement that we have been understood. Many times, however, when we interact with another person, we want something from them.

For example, we might directly ask someone for something such as a pay rise, or permission to take a holiday; we may unconsciously word our conversation in such a way as to gain approval or reassurance from a respected friend or colleague. When 'gossiping' we may impart sensational information, seeking a reaction and additional information to further the scandal and for our amusement. When we complain to someone, we are seeking to be understood, even empathized with, and assured that action will be taken. We may wish to put on a show to demonstrate that we are more knowledgeable than someone who has been bothering us. We may wish to boast about our lives to score a point from someone who has annoyed us by doing the same.

When we express a need for a particular response from someone, consciously or unconsciously, we give the locus of power to the other person, thereby giving them control of our present wellbeing. We move the locus of power in the conversation towards the other person when we allow ourselves to be emotionally attached to that person's response. The more emotionally attached we are, the more external our locus of control, and the more we invite the other person to influence our thoughts, feelings and behaviours.

For example, if we are asking for a particular day of holiday and we really want this day off, we are emotionally attached to the outcome. To ensure we get the outcome we want, we might find ourselves asking for it in a wheedling voice, using emotive language. We might adopt an inferior body language when we speak to the person who has the power to grant us what we want and we might offer them something in return, perhaps more of a compromise than is required. If we have a day of holiday to take but we are not concerned about when it is, we are more likely to just ask for a day off. We are not attached to the outcome; if we cannot have that day, then we will take another. The power dynamics in these two situations are very different, despite being the same request.

When we are attached to the outcome, if it is positive we feel elated but, if the answer is 'no', we can fall into dejection. Our emotional state is at the mercy of another. The person saying 'no' may have good reasons to do so but we are unlikely to see this; instead we see it as a personal slight. Here, our locus of control has become more external. When we are unattached to the outcome, we are more able to see the reasons behind the answer and are less affected by it.

When we seek approval and reassurance from others, rather than believing in ourselves, we again shift our locus of control externally. If our self-worth depends on compliments from others, we put ourselves wholly in their power. A negative comment, or even a lack of praise, can feel like failure. If we feel as though someone is putting us down, we may in reality be simply attaching an emotional significance to their response and choosing to feel inferior.

If we feel inferior, then we have pushed our locus of control externally and allowed ourselves to be affected by another's words and actions. If we look to ourselves and recognize our own self-worth, then it will not matter what anyone says or does.

Some of us will give away the locus of power easily in our communications. Others will keep it towards themselves so that they are more in control of the situation (a little like keeping our cards close to our chest). This will depend on such things as personality and previous experience.

We can improve our resilience by observing our own behaviour in all our interactions. Collecting information like this allows us to spot patterns and, eventually, make our responses conscious rather than unconscious.

There are many reasons why we might shift the locus of power towards others and, therefore, away from the Self. Exploring the reasons why you interact in the way that you do will improve your understanding and lead to more conscious communication.

Power dynamics are complex. There will always be both a balance and an exchange of power in human interaction. Sometimes we must give away some of the power for a useful interaction to take place. The key is to raise our awareness and consciously choose what is appropriate, rather than acting out of unconscious need. Remember, no one can take the locus of power in an interaction unless you give it to them.

In the same way, we have a responsibility to not abuse our power. In conversation, some people are very skilled at perceiving when they have been given the locus of power and they can make a conscious decision as to how to respond. If this is not done with integrity or for the greatest good of all concerned, conflict may well arise from the situation.

For example, if the employer in the scenario discussed at the beginning of this chapter recognizes our need and decides not to grant it anyway for no sound reason, then she is abusing the power dynamic in the relationship. Pulling the locus of relational power towards the Self can feel good. It can make us feel powerful. It will, however, ultimately damage the relationship and can lead to its breakdown.

Being truly powerful is being aware of power dynamics but not abusing them. It is remaining unaffected by the efforts of others to manipulate them. It is being aware of, but not advertising, our emotional need and, in addressing that need in ourselves, we can balance the locus of power in our interactions.

In conclusion, understanding and mastering our part in the 'great dance' of communication is both enlightening and empowering. When we recognize where the locus of power sits, we can move it towards ourselves or towards others to accomplish what we want to achieve. Learning to balance the power dynamic in our relationships helps us develop healthier, stronger interactions. When we are in conflict with others, being aware of the locus of power and its effect on our communications will help us manage the situation. In Part 3 you will find tools and techniques to help observe your power, balance the locus and manage conflict situations.

Part 2
CORE SKILLS

This part of the book outlines the core skills required to get the most benefit from using the Resilience Toolkit. We have distilled these skills from both modern and ancient practices across the globe. Here, we will teach you to apply the knowledge of self-awareness that you have gained in Part 1, and prepare you to use the tools in Part 3.

8

Observation and choice

To acquire knowledge, one must study; but to acquire wisdom, one must observe.

Marilyn vos Savant

In Part 1 of this book we have explored, in some depth, several concepts which help to explain our human responses and patterns of behaviour. These have included conditioning, emotions, universal laws, shadow work, survival archetypes and the locus of power in relationships. In this part, we will show you how to apply all that you have learned about those concepts. The purpose of this is to overcome resistance to change – to encourage evolution rather than repetition of negative patterns.

As we have previously suggested, simply raising *awareness* of these concepts is often enough to effect progress. However, we need to wake up to what is going on within us and live more consciously. We do this by *observing* our internal processes and consciously *choosing* our thoughts, feelings and behaviours. This replaces the old model where we automatically react. Imagine the energy that is required to live in your emotions and to act immediately as a result of them. Now you can use that energy for something of your choosing.

We are going to show you how to observe and then harness your power to consciously choose. You will learn how to apply this core skill to all the theory from Part 1. We have discussed the concepts individually. However, in reality, they do not operate separately at all. Our conditioning, core beliefs and shadow are always present, influencing our thoughts, feelings and behaviours. Survival archetypes will always step in when we are fearful, and the universal laws overarch everything. You will see the interconnectedness as we describe examples below.

'Observation and choice' in practice

We begin this process with *observation*. Within the field of psychotherapy, there is a recognized part of our psyche which is referred to as the Observer Self.[1] This is the part of us that can report that something made us feel sad or angry or upset. It is not the part of us that actually does the feeling. It is the one that collects the data.

When connecting with this part of the Self and making the distinction between the observer and the feeler, we can learn to observe and detach from our emotions. When we do not feel the emotions, we are unbiased in our recording of the information. We realize that *we are not the emotion*; we are separate from it and, therefore, the information is more accurate and balanced. The Observer Self can stand back and report the emotions that are at play, without becoming consumed by them. This is liberating.

It is important to remember that, when we stand in the shoes of the Observer Self, *we do not judge*. We simply watch and collect the information; we observe ourselves and our responses to certain situations without analysis and, preferably, without thought.

When we cultivate the ability to observe these thoughts and emotions within ourselves, we make them conscious. In other, words we become aware of them. The awareness of these processes provides us with much useful information. When we foster the habit of connection with the observing part of the psyche, we can begin to see cycles and patterns in our own thoughts, feelings and behaviours. This is the prerequisite to harnessing the power to *choose*.

Do I repeat? Or do I take a different path this time?

We can do this with kindness towards ourselves. Repeating is easy and feels comfortable, because the familiar cycle of thoughts, feelings and behaviour is already established in our neural pathways. Taking a different path is unfamiliar and evokes fear. Journeys that involve uncertainty are considered perilous by the psyche. This is why we unconsciously block ourselves.

The next time that you find yourself in a situation where something in the external environment has created an emotional change within you, you can engage your Observer Self. As soon as you feel that change take place, for example a churning stomach, a tight chest, the hairs standing up on the back of your neck, *press pause*.

Take your awareness to a physical thing, for example your breathing or your heartbeat. This helps you to become present in the situation. When you are present, you are less likely to be influenced by past events or future imaginings.

Now step into the shoes of your Observer Self. This is the part of you that collects all of the detail of the situation so that you will be able to recount it later. It does not judge. It simply watches and notices everything – how your thoughts, feelings and behaviours are being influenced by your conditioning, your shadow, your archetypes, the universal laws and the locus of power.

As you stand in these shoes, you are able to stand back from the emotion that has been generated. You can watch the situation play out and notice the processes involved. These are both *internal* (what is going on for you) and *external* (what is going on for others). You are privy to the current situation, however, only through your own lens. You are *not* privy to how others are dealing with it, and therefore you must understand that their behaviour is not always about you.

Remember that we cannot change the behaviour of other parties; we can only *observe* and *choose* our own responses. If we perceive that someone is upsetting us, it is *we* who are upset. The behaviour of another may be entirely abhorrent, but in recovery, the *only* important thing is *our* response. It is the only thing that we can control.

Once you have collected all the information, you are afforded the opportunity to choose:

- You can observe and do nothing.
- You can allow old behavioural responses to play out.
- You can choose new conscious responses.

Sometimes you will let old patterns repeat because it serves you. Sometimes you will choose new alternatives. Sometimes you will choose to do nothing. You will gain valuable information either way.

What matters is that your choice is conscious.

> Here is step-by-step summary for 'observation and choice.'
>
> 1. Press *pause*.
>
> 2. Become present.
>
> 3. Step into the shoes of the Observer Self.
>
> 4. Witness *all* aspects of the situation.
>
> 5. Consciously choose your response.

Overcoming resistance

When we are embarking on a journey towards self-improvement, growth or enlightenment, we often find ourselves blocked. This is widely known as *resistance.*

When we resist, rather than applying the principle of 'observation and choice' we stay with our automatic responses. This differs from a conscious choice to repeat, change or not to act. It is unconscious and triggered by fear. As we have said before, fear arises when we feel we are going to lose something. This drives negative projection and, in turn, resistant behaviour. We know we are experiencing resistance when we hear ourselves affirming the reasons why we cannot move forward.

Examples of this internal narrative include:

- I've always been like this. I can't change now.
- I can't because of what happened to me.
- It's not going to work for me.
- I'm too tired to start something new.
- I can't afford it.
- If I do this I might lose out.
- I don't understand.
- I don't know where to start.
- I might get hurt.
- I can't do this on my own; I need help.
- It won't change the outcome; xyz will still happen.
- I'm fine the way things are; I don't actually want to change.
- I don't know what I'm doing; I'll never master it.
- My family/friends/colleagues won't like it.
- If I change things, I'm afraid that xyz will happen.
- I have enough to deal with; I couldn't possibly do this as well.
- I have no will power and will never be able to see it through.
- I can't change another person's behaviour; it is not my fault that they are doing this to me.

If you look closely at all of these reasons for not moving forward, you will be able to attribute each of them to at least one of the survival archetypes. You may also be able to attribute them to other aspects of the psyche learned about in Part 1. When you hear resistance such as this in your responses, the first thing to do is to activate the Observer Self.

You are now aware that the thought of your moving forward has provoked the response of fear. Acknowledge its presence. *Fear is your friend and protector. Sit with it in gratitude.*

Now you can ask yourself:

- What do I have to *lose* from moving forward?
- What are my attachments to the way that things are now?

When you see resistance, the key is to acknowledge it. Then you are free to consciously choose your response.

Resistance can occur as a result of learned behaviour. In Chapter 2, we explored the theory that we each have a unique internal model of the world, which is a product of our conditioning: our parenting, life experiences and genetic make-up. We explained that, as children, we learn and develop through the consequences of our behaviour. Those patterns of behaviour, which keep us from harm and result in our getting what we need (e.g. love, attention, food, approval), are processed and integrated internally. As such, they extend into adulthood and, ultimately, become habit. They are also responsible for creating much of our circumstance. Some patterns of behaviour that are learned in childhood are no longer helpful in our adult lives. They create unwanted situations and must be replaced with something that better serves us.

We know how we should be addressing a problem, but changing our behaviour feels uncomfortable. We have behaved in a certain way for our whole life and it has got us far. Besides, we have no frame of reference as to how to behave otherwise.

For example, a person who was praised as a child for finishing all the food on her plate at mealtimes may, as an adult, continue to feel the need to eat more food than is necessary to satisfy her hunger for praise. This, along with a host of other reasons, may contribute to her becoming overweight. Although the obvious answer is to stop eating when she is full (even if this means leaving food on her plate), this feels uncomfortable and goes against a lifetime of habit which, as far as the child who processed the behaviour is concerned, has got her this far unscathed.

When children trip and fall, they often look around to see who has noticed. If no one has, they may pick themselves up and run on. If an adult has noticed, they often cry or shout to attract attention. When adults respond by giving comfort, the child's behaviour may be adopted as an appropriate response to any injury as it achieved the desired effect. In adults, this behaviour may still be present but age-adapted in some way. Often, this leads to an unconscious attachment to a problem or condition.

We sometimes experience resistance when we perceive that the desired outcome may result in the removal of something which we do not want to lose. For example, a person who has been cared for through a short-term illness may not want to lose that connection. This can result in an attachment to illness and pain.

When you notice unhealthy learned patterns in yourself, once again activate your Observer Self.

Resistance can also be affected by our relationships with others. Remember that you are part of a complex network of relationships and you will have many roles. You may be child, parent, sibling, partner, friend, colleague, patient and so on. Clearly, our behaviour affects those around us, and the locus of power in relationships can compound our problem and compromise and limit our choices. We need to recognize this and incorporate it into our learning, rather than using it as a reason not to continue.

This is perhaps best illustrated using the example of a person with a terminal diagnosis. In our experience, people sometimes struggle to tell loved ones about their condition. This is usually because they are afraid of upsetting them and worry about how they will react. Everyone involved has high emotions and expresses them in different ways. Everyone is wary of how others are feeling. In fact, we *never* know how someone else is feeling; we can only project. We never really know a person fully; we only know the version of them that we have created based on our model of the world.

We project in two ways: how we would feel, or how we think our version of them would feel. As usual, these beliefs lead to thoughts, which lead to emotions, which, in turn, affect behaviours. We believe that a person will respond in a certain way; this affects our thoughts and feelings about how they will react, which affects how we behave towards them.

When you feel yourself modifying your behaviour in this way, activate your Observer Self.

There will be resistance throughout the process of cultivating resilience because it is part of our nature. We must observe it, acknowledge it and move through it in a conscious way. Regardless of how uncomfortable it makes you feel, ALWAYS ask yourself what you are gaining from the negative situation. You can then utilize the power of choice to generate a more positive outcome. Remember that any backward steps along the journey are part of the process and resistance is expected. Your Observer Self is a great teacher. Cultivate the habit of observing your own processes as they happen, and you will become conscious in all situations.

9

Language

The limits of my language mean the limits of my world.

Ludwig Wittgenstein

We discussed earlier how we unconsciously express our emotions and intentions with tone and non-verbal communication. We are now going to talk about the *words* that we use towards ourselves and others. In this chapter, we are going to teach you how to use language for the benefit of all. The core skill here is the *conscious choice of words*.

In Chapter 7, we outlined many of the reasons for entering into communication with another person or group of people. We explained that we do this to express a need, impart information, or because we are seeking a particular response. When we decide to express ourselves, we formulate what we are going to say by selecting from the vocabulary that we have stored in our memory. The words we choose are based on our needs. These may be conscious or unconscious. Our unconscious needs are always communicated non-verbally, whether we like it or not. This means that we may be saying one thing with our words while communicating something entirely different with our body language and tone. In her Warrior Goddess Training Programme, HeatherAsh Amara describes these as 'contaminated messages'.[1]

The level of consciousness in choosing our words varies, depending on the situation. Some people speak with more conscious awareness than others. Those are usually the people who have mastered the core skill of observation and conscious choice (Chapter 8).

As we described in Chapter 2, the things that were said to us during childhood contribute to our core beliefs about the Self and are, therefore, partly responsible for our conditioning.

We have all heard the phrase 'Sticks and stones may break my bones, but words can never hurt me'. This is not true. In fact, words not only hurt us – they shape and define us.

Words are incredibly powerful. They are either poison or medicine and, when we have learned the core skill of language, we can choose which. We have all felt the balm of calming words in a crisis or words of love and appreciation when we have felt undervalued. Conversely, we have felt the sting of someone telling us an uncomfortable truth about the Self that we did not wish to acknowledge. Here, we will share some basic principles of structuring sentences and phrases which aim to have the greatest impact on the listener. Remember that the listener includes the Self.

Before you pick up your phone to text, comment on social media, send an email, make knee-jerk comments on the phone or in an altercation, or admonish yourself, *press pause*.

Ask yourself the following question: 'What is my intention?' Listen to the answer.

- Is it to judge so that I am less judged?
- Is it to compare myself to someone else so that I know that I am where I should be?
- Is it to teach someone a lesson that they can learn without my intervention?
- Is it the joy of passing on a nugget of gossip or a secret?

There will never be no consequences. We tattoo ourselves and others with words. Most damaging or healing are the words we use towards ourselves.

Speaking to the Self

Reframing

We are constantly processing information. To do this we use *thought*. When we examine them, thoughts can be expressed in words. With the use of our thoughts, we create an *internal narrative*. This is a stream of verbal thinking which affirms our understanding of the way things are.

In therapy, when someone presents with an outmoded behaviour that no longer suits them, we ask, 'What is the internal narrative here? What are you saying to yourself?'

We speak to the Self all the time. A *mantra* is something that we say to ourselves on a regular basis. The regular repetition of a message is known as *affirmation*. Affirmation is one way of driving a message into the subconscious, thereby creating *belief*.

Consider the power of *words*, *mantras*, and *affirmation* on our core beliefs about the Self. Imagine the positive changes that would arise from applying the concept of *observation and conscious choice* here.

Ask yourself the following questions:

- **'What do I say to myself every day?'** Phrases might include: *I never learn, I'm so tired, I'm no good at this, I'm so fat, I'm so stupid, I never have any money, I'm so busy, I have no time, I'm so disorganized, I'm so rubbish.*
- **'What is it that I need to hear every day?'** This is where you would use the core skill of language to change those mantras into phrases like: *I'm always learning, I'm getting better at this, I am healthy and well, I have the power to choose what I eat, I am capable, I have enough money, I have plenty of energy, I can choose to rest when I need to, I have purpose, I am valuable.*

This is *reframing*. It is a vital skill. Use it when the answers to the two above questions are not aligned.

Reframing was first described by Aaron T. Beck in the 1960s as part of his cognitive therapy.[2] It was expanded upon in a therapeutic setting by Richard Bandler and John Grinder in the 1970s.[3] They developed Neurolinguistic Programming (NLP), which is an approach to communication and personal growth in talking therapy. NLP has since been widely used as a powerful language tool in many industries, including motivational coaching, politics, business, sales and psychotherapy.

Positive reframing refers to changing the wording of a sentence or narrative from negative to positive. When we positively reframe our mantras, we affect our core beliefs. When positively reframe our core beliefs; we positively affect our thoughts and narratives, our resulting emotions and, in turn, our behaviours.

As discussed in Chapter 3, this positively affects our body chemistry. There are specific step-by-step tools for reframing thoughts and core beliefs in Part 3.

Structuring suggestions

Many talking therapies are suggestion based. The therapist must structure any suggestions that are made in such a way as to have the most positive impact. With that in mind, applying the following techniques for structuring suggestions can be extremely useful when speaking to the Self.

- **Use positive language.** It is widely understood that the unconscious mind is not receptive to words such as 'no' and 'not'. Rather than using uncertain language (such as 'may' or 'might'), use affirmative words such as 'will'.
  - o For example, if you are using suggestion to address tiredness, instead of using a phrase like 'I am *not* tired' or 'I have *no* fatigue', try 'I have enough energy to perform my tasks' or 'I have the power to choose to rest when I need to.' Instead of saying 'I *might* manage to stop smoking', try 'I *will* stop smoking.'

- **Keep instructions simple and sentences at a low word level.** The unconscious mind processes most efficiently when given one suggestion at a time.
  - For example, instead of saying 'I will eat food that is healthy for me and exercise regularly', try 'I will eat food that is healthy for me', followed by 'I will exercise regularly.'

- **Use emotive words.** If you want to drive the message home, you need to use words which suggest positive emotional outcomes.
  - For example, rather than saying 'When I speak publicly I will be confident and look like I know what I'm doing', try 'When I speak publicly, I will *ooze confidence and radiate expertise.'*

Learning to reframe our mantras, thoughts and core beliefs is hugely empowering. You can use language to choose how to think, feel and behave.

Having discussed how we speak to the Self, we will now explore the words we choose when speaking to others.

Speaking to others

If we want our interaction with others to have maximum positive impact, we should apply the same principles to those communications as we apply when speaking to the Self. We can use our skills in observation and then utilize our power to choose by reframing and rewording what we want to say.

Here are two further language tools which are extremely useful when communicating with others. The first has its roots in NLP.

Three powerful words

We would like to share three powerful words. We learned about these in our usual line of work by reading David McDonnell's book *How to Communicate Basically Brilliantly with Patients.*[4]

Those words are *when, but* and *aware*:

1. McDonnell shows how the word 'when' allows patients to imagine a positive future. We might use it when talking to patients who are worried and anxious – for example *'When* you are feeling better' or *'When* your pain is reduced.' You can apply this in a non-clinical setting – for example *'When* my family is reconciled' or *'When* I pass my driving test.'

2. The word 'but' cancels out everything that was said before it. When talking to patients about treatment, we must be careful where in the sentence we put this word. Any positive messages we put before it will be lost. Any negative messages after it will be reinforced. So rather than 'This medication is really effective, *but* it may make you feel a bit sick', we say 'This may make you feel a bit sick *but* it is a really effective medication.' In a non-clinical setting, rather than 'I love you, *but* I find your recent behaviour really annoying', we might prefer to say 'I find your recent behaviour really annoying, *but* I love you.'

3. The word 'aware' helps to alert the person to whom you are speaking to what you are saying. It raises their awareness. We might use this in health promotion. Rather than saying 'You really should stop smoking because it causes cancer', we might say 'Were you aware that, *when* you stop smoking, your risk of getting lots of different cancers will go down?' This empowers the person you are talking to. In a non-clinical setting, rather than saying, or shouting, 'TIDY YOUR BEDROOM!' we might say 'Are you aware that, if you make your bedroom a lovely organized space, you will feel good when you spend time there?'

The Thank You Technique

The second language skill for use when speaking to others is our own. It is called the Thank You Technique. This is extremely useful in situations of conflict and draws on everything that we have discussed about self-awareness.

We can now recognize that we are viewing every situation through our own unique lens. Having gained a good under-standing of universal law, shadow work, pain body, survival archetypes and locus of power, we know that our responses to all events are based on our own model of the world. Here, every time someone says something that upsets us, we say 'thank you'.

The Thank You Technique works in three ways:

1. It helps us to stand back and observe the emotion generated by the event, rather than being consumed by it. Rather than replying with an emotion-fuelled response, we say, *'Thank you* for those comments.' This breaks the, otherwise inevi-table, chain of events – we react, they react, repeating the cycle until we are in conflict. The Thank You Technique prevents this escalation. The technique is useful when we are faced with aggression. An aggressor will be expecting certain responses to their behaviour. Saying 'thank you' does not allow them those responses and therefore does not feed that aggression.

2. It creates space for us to examine where, within us, we are being prompted to work. To assess which part of the Self has been uncomfortably provoked. We are actually saying 'thank you' to the universe for the experience. We can recognize why what the person has said has upset us, and which parts of the Self are being reflected, or which parts of our shadow are being highlighted. We are saying 'thank you' because we are *grateful for the opportunity for growth.*

3. It helps us consciously process feedback. When we receive feedback, we should be thankful for it and the lessons it offers us. No one likes criticism, but it is worth remembering that we only react strongly to feedback that we believe is true. If we believe it because we know that we need to improve or

change, then we can *thank* the universe for the pointer. If we believe it is true because of an unhealthy negative core belief, reflection or shadow, then we can *thank* the universe for the opportunity to recognize this and do the work.

It is worth remembering that compliments can be as difficult to process as criticism. This is because they truly challenge our negative core beliefs about the Self. However uncomfortable you feel, remember that, by accepting a compliment, you are really complimenting the person that gave it to you. They have seen something of themselves that is pleasing reflected in you. Use the Thank You Technique here, too. *Thank* them for the positive feedback, and *thank* the universe for the opportunity to explore why it made you so uncomfortable.

When we use this technique, we must watch our tone. We must say 'thank you' sincerely even when we are annoyed because, when we project our gratitude, we are activating the Universal Law of Attraction. Saying 'thank you' with sarcasm is not conducive to progress.

Although much of communication takes place non-verbally, we must appreciate the power of words and learn how to use them with integrity and for the good of all.

10

Breathing consciously

For breath is life, so if you breathe well you will live long on earth.

Sanskrit proverb

Breath is synonymous with life. It is the first thing we do after we are born and the last thing that we do before we die. When we are in crisis, we tell ourselves to 'breathe'. We know the importance of breathing and, yet, we often forget to make our breathing a conscious tool to improve our wellbeing.

The connection between breath and spirit is recognized across all cultures. This is affirmed in the Latin word *spiritus*, which means spirit, courage, vigour and breath. In Sanskrit, the word *prana* describes energy and spirit, but also respiration and breath. In Arabic, the word for spirit is associated with air. There are countless breathing rituals and exercises which exist for the purpose of spiritual and meditative practice. In traditional shamanism, the spirit is believed to enter the body with the first breath and leave with the last. Sharing of breath with all living things is further affirmation that we are all connected.

The ability to *breathe consciously* is a core skill and a prerequisite to improving resilience.

We have both reported various incidents in our daily lives where we remember feeling that we 'forgot to breathe'. This is because, when we are under pressure, we may fall into the habit of taking tiny gulping breaths that give us the minimum amount of gaseous exchange for us to function. We do not need *only* to function. We need to be fully nourished. We are far more efficient if we give breathing our attention.

It is widely known that rapid breathing, or hyperventilation, causes 'blowing off' of the normal amounts of carbon dioxide in the lungs, reducing levels in the blood. It is the building up of that carbon dioxide that drives us to breathe. Removing the drive to breathe causes panic attacks which create further rapid breathing.

When we exercise to the point of exhaustion, we may find ourselves leaning on a surface with our arms to help us get our breath back. This is because the muscles in the top of the shoulders and neck act as accessory muscles for breathing when fixed in this way. It encourages large volumes of airflow into the tops of the lungs, helping us to recover. It is a common human habit to utilize the upper lobes of the lungs rather than to breathe deeply, using the diaphragm. This type of shallow breathing is not efficient. When you consider the above fact, remember also that many of us are regularly propped up on our elbows, squinting into a laptop screen, fixing our accessory muscles. Are you doing this right now?

When we are stressed or upset, we can feel like our shoulders are up by our ears. Consciously drawing the shoulder blades down and together, relaxing the neck and face, releases the accessory muscles and allows for deeper, more nourishing breaths.

We are not alone in our appreciation of the benefits of conscious breathing. Jon Kabat-Zinn's mindfulness-based stress reduction (MBSR) programme[1] is now widely taught in hospitals and medical establishments throughout the Western world. Conscious breathing is an incredibly useful tool in achieving mindfulness and meditation; however, some of our exercises use the physical act of breathing *alone* to promote positive change.

The physiological and psychological effects of slow breathing exercises are well documented. Controlling breath has been shown to affect heart rate and brain waves. Experiences of increased comfort, relaxation, pleasantness, vigour and alertness and reduced symptoms of anxiety, depression, anger and confusion are reported.[2]

Diaphragmatic breathing stimulates the vagal nerve, which down-regulates the fight/flight chemical reaction. This is known as 'the relaxation response'.[3]

Conscious breathing

We will now describe the essential core skill of *conscious breathing*:

1. Sit up straight, drop your shoulders allowing your shoulder blades to fall down and come together. Unclench your jaw and relax your face.
2. Take your awareness to your *breathing*.
3. Give it no thought, just *conscious awareness*.
4. Notice your chest and abdomen rising and falling.
5. Allow your breath to slow and deepen.
6. Follow the air right to the bottoms of your lungs.
7. Notice where, in your body, you feel your *heartbeat*.
8. Know that your breath connects to your *heart*.
9. Notice the *physical sensations* that you feel.
10. Become aware of feelings of calm, relaxation and wellbeing that arise within you as you continue to breathe slowly and comfortably.

Do not apply any thinking to this exercise, only *awareness of sensation*.

All the meditation techniques we teach begin with an awareness of breathing. This kind of approach has its roots in Buddhism. We follow up that awareness with a deepening and lengthening of the breath, especially the outbreath which promotes physical relaxation in the body. This allows us to enter an altered state of awareness, where we are better able to access our psychological processes.

If breath and life are synonymous, perhaps one who masters breath can master life itself.

11

Visualization

The clearer you are when visualizing your dreams, the brighter the spotlight will be to lead you on the right path.

Gail Lynne Goodwin

Visualization *(noun)*: The act of forming a picture of somebody/something in your mind.

Visualization is an essential core skill required to use our resilience toolbox. With many of the tools we teach, especially the guided meditations, we are often aiming to set a scene. We are creating a picture to work with (e.g., imagine a beautiful waterfall). Sometimes we are aiming to recall memory (e.g., take yourself back to your first day at school). The more clear and vivid the image, the more effective the exercise will be. We are aiming to create an image which is easy for our subconscious mind to work with. This reduces resistance. It prevents our conscious mind from stepping in and telling us that we cannot see a believable picture and, therefore, we cannot progress any further.

Although the title of this chapter is 'Visualization', we are actually talking about creating a picture which is acceptable to the subconscious mind. To do this, we must, in fact, use *all* of our senses.

The visual, auditory and kinaesthetic (VAK) model, first introduced by Barbe[1] and later expanded upon by Fleming,[2] suggests that some people are better able to learn and process with the use of one sense rather than another. This model is discussed in more detail in Chapter 15. In fact, we all learn using a combination of *all* of our senses, but the extent to which we utilize each one varies from person to person.

People who describe themselves as visual learners will use phrases like 'I see what you are saying', 'Picture this' and 'I can't see that happening.' They find it easy to picture events and recall and describe settings.

Auditory people will say 'I hear you', 'That sounds good to me' and 'That's music to my ears.' They will always remember what was said to them at key events and often have an affinity with music.

Kinaesthetic people will use visceral phrases and sentences like 'my gut feeling', 'It didn't feel right' and 'He made my skin crawl.' They will be sensitive to changes of mood picked up in the non-verbal communication of others as they will *feel* it in their body.

Olfactory people will be very connected to taste and smell and may use language like 'I smell a rat' or 'It left a nasty taste in my mouth.' We have all experienced the evocative effect of taste and smell on memory and emotion.

We are all capable of using all of our senses for processing but, in practice, each of us tends to lean towards a predominant one.

In the workshops we have done together and with others, we have come to learn that Karen works very well kinaesthetically. This means that she predominantly sets the scene through feeling what is there. Chrissie has a bias towards auditory processing. This means that when working in this way, sounds and words are often more significant. Once again, we must use our core skill of *observe and choose.* Although we are being asked to visualize, we become aware of and accept which senses we work best with and learn how this helps us to set the scene. For example, in recalling a childhood birthday party, Karen might ask herself 'What am I feeling?' whereas Chrissie might ask, 'What can I hear?'

When we first begin to introduce this type of work in our workshops, we are often met with some frustration on the part of our delegates – people who have come to learn and are wholly compliant in the process but feel that their stumbling block is that they just cannot visualize. This frustration serves only to compound the problem, as they feel that, without this skill, they will never move forward.

Taking the person who perceives that they have the least amount of visualization skill, we ask them to close their eyes and describe the front of their house. Within seconds, the words that they are using are accompanied by hand gestures which *draw out* the shape of the windows and porch. They are visualizing. The pictures that we see do not always appear like postcards or photographs. The best thing to do, if you are worried that you are not seeing images, is to relax and simply know that they are there.

When we are visualizing during an exercise, we must intensify the image with information from our other senses. Such information can provide important insights. For example, begin to imagine a really pleasant day at the seaside when you were a child. You might be able to visualize the sand, water, bucket and spade, but the image would be greatly enhanced by the smell of fish and chips and candyfloss and the cry of the seagulls. This would also serve to evoke emotion and memory. The more that we practise these skills, the more effective our work will be.

In shamanic journeying, we are not given guidance as to what to 'see'. We are asked to accept and trust what comes. We are better able to achieve this when we are practised at visualization.

Below are some exercises to improve visualization skills:

1. Take a simple object from your surroundings. Hold it in your hands. Examine it closely, taking in every piece of information that it has to offer you. Do not forget about your other senses.
2. Now put down the object and close your eyes. Try to picture it in your mind's eye, just exactly as it was when you were looking at it. If it begins to fade, repeat the process.

3. Now put the object out of sight and write or speak a detailed description of it. Know that, without visualization of the object, you would not be able to describe it.

4. Alternatively, put the object out of sight and take a pencil and paper. Begin to recall the object and draw it exactly as it appears to you in your mind's eye. The quality of your artwork is not important here. Just know that object is out of sight and so the image that you produced came only from your visualization.

---

1. Now try the above exercise with a more detailed image, such as a photograph or several different objects. Remember to use your mind's eye to create a detailed description or image, rather than verbally recalling what was there.

2. Now create a mental image of a simple object without a visual reference – for example an apple. It is easy to remember what an apple looks like, but you cannot *describe* your particular apple without visualization. You can also draw your apple.

3. Now try creating a more complex imagined image. Take a scene from a story that you have read but not seen adapted on to a screen. Imagine the backdrop in detail. Visualize the characters in your story. Be creative. See them as clearly as you can. Utilize your other senses. Become involved in the story. Allow your emotions to come alive.

4. Now describe the scene so as to pass on every physical detail for another person to be able to visualize it too.

5. You can also draw the scene. Focus on the details; the parts that tell the story. Try to get the message of what is happening across in your picture. Again, do not worry about the quality of your art; just know that you drew those things because you were able to visualize them.

The purpose of doing these exercises is twofold. Firstly, repetitive practice leads to skill enhancement, and, secondly, describing and drawing your visions in detail is affirmation that you are doing it right!

Many of our tools require a degree of visualization. You do not have to be a particular type of person or possess any skill that is not common to all of us. You simply need to understand that there are no rules when visualizing. You must trust that however things appear to you is exactly right for you.

12

Cultivating stillness with meditation

The mind is like water. When it is turbulent, it is difficult to see. When it is calm, everything becomes clear.

Prasad Mahes

This chapter explains the value of stillness, which must precede every one of our resilience tools and, indeed, every action we undertake. Before the curtain rises in the theatre, there is a moment of stillness in the performers and the audience, a moment of anticipation. Learning to cultivate that moment brings lasting benefits for our physical and mental health. Meditation is the best way to achieve that stillness and is a core resilience skill. This chapter discusses the importance of meditation and demonstrates the science that proves its benefit. It also describes how to prepare for meditation; to prepare our space and ourselves.

Modern life is always hectic. We race from one meeting or appointment to another. We squeeze as much as we can into every waking minute. Even when we do have a spare moment, our minds are never still. We may feel a need to be busy at all times, craving distraction and entertainment. When we are doing, we are not still. It is in *stillness* that we can reflect. Just as a still pool of water reflects a perfect image of the Self, when we are still, we are able to reflect for ourselves and others. When we are still, we become a mirror so that we and those around us can find our own answers. When we are still in our interaction with others, we can stay out of the way of their progress. If we can learn to quieten the chatter of our thoughts and be still, our own answers come to us in silence. It is important to learn the value of stillness. Consider also that stillness precedes right action.

A gymnast must first achieve a moment of perfect stillness before showcasing what appears to be the impossible. During communication or even conflict, there are small spaces between the exchanges of sentences and expressions of thought where it is possible to achieve stillness. When we harness these moments, time appears to slow down and we are able to calmly and perfectly deliver the information required for the greater good. This is because the information comes from a place of deeper knowing that we can only access when we are still.

Imagine that you are on a long journey. You must transport a bucket of water from the beginning of the journey to your destination. When the ground is rocky, making you lose your footing, or when there is adverse weather, the water slops from one side of the bucket to the other and back again, repeatedly, until balance is reached. When you stop and breathe, the turbulence eventually subsides. When you have achieved stillness, not only can you see right to the bottom of the bucket, you can also see yourself reflected in the still water.

Meditation is an ancient practice in which we can train the Self to increase concentration and attention, cultivating stillness of the mind. It has been practised for thousands of years and in many different cultures and religions. It can be said that during meditation we experience an *altered state of awareness*. This is somewhere between sleep and fully alert. We experience this kind of altered state when we are waking up in the morning; we have heard the alarm and decide we will have five more minutes. The next time we look at the clock, half an hour has passed. We can hear the noises of our home and the start of the day but we are in a half-wakeful state and our perception of time is affected. Many of us have also experienced this while driving. We reach our destination with no recollection of the journey itself. A similar altered state of awareness is experienced in hypnosis. A hypnotherapist will guide a person deeper into trance with the use of suggestion.

It is important to make the distinction between *meditation* and *mindfulness*. Being mindful is choosing to be in the present moment; all our thoughts are solely on the now, truly immersed in what we are doing. Being aware of our thoughts and emotions as our Observer Self with no judgement. This means being consciously aware of everything but not thinking about it. We do not need to alter our state of awareness to become mindful.

Meditation is the habitual practice of a chosen technique to still the mind, calming the unfocused, and often futile, repetitive thoughts that fill our awareness. Meditation usually results in an altered state of awareness. The goal is to centre the mind on to a single thing to cultivate stillness and increase our focus, leaving our mind clear and our emotions tranquil. Meditation can be a vehicle to a mindful state, and there is a style of meditation called 'mindfulness meditation'. There are, however, many different meditation styles and techniques which do not require us to be in the present moment. For example, regression and past and future meditations.

We describe a selection of these techniques below in the hope that you find a method that suits you. The most important thing is that you try them. This is a vital core skill.

In Part 3 you will find many guided meditations, each with a specific purpose, for you to try. This is the easiest way to get started; record yourself speaking the meditations slowly and calmly; your mobile phone is ideal for this. You can then guide yourself in meditation whenever you want.

Our website has audios of the guided meditations if you would prefer to listen to someone else. Chrissie's voice has been likened to listening to melted chocolate! Remember, it is not about being an expert meditator who can levitate; it is about learning a new skill, and that takes practice. Weave this practice into your daily life.

Types of meditation

- **Guided meditations**: these aim to talk you through the process of getting into a meditative state. The guidance is provided by an experienced practitioner, in person or digitally. It is ideal for beginners as a starting point.

- **Scripted meditations**: these guided meditations have a specific purpose. Within them are metaphors and structured suggestions. Listening to a prerecorded meditation to achieve a specific goal such as sleep, addressing anxiety, cultivating a healthy lifestyle or improving performance. We can listen to meditations that take us into the past, such as rescuing our inner child, or the future such as visualizing a desired outcome. This process can also be described as self-hypnosis.

- **Mindfulness meditation**: this is open-minded or open awareness meditation (also known as mindful meditation). It is a Buddhist practice. Mindfulness meditation involves allowing the thoughts in our conscious mind to rise up and then fade away. We observe them without judging or allowing them to take our focus. This is easily accessible as it can be unguided and without audio.

- **Focused meditation**: this is also a good starting place for beginners, and, again, it is an easy one to practise unguided, as the technique is about focusing on one thing to quiet the inner voice and the hundreds of thoughts in our head. Popular examples of what people focus on are their breathing or the flame of a candle. The purpose of the focus is to fix our attention and prevent our thoughts from wandering. As they do this, we can gently bring our attention back to the object of our focus. The next step in this meditation is to remove the object of our focus, leaving a void (this is challenging).

- **Movement meditation**: this refers to any techniques where activity is used as the focus for our attention. There are elements of movement meditation in many cultures. The beauty of this technique is how expressive it can be. You can dance, jump or beat a drum – whatever resonates with you. Walking meditation is a popular example. In the traditional form of this method, participants walk clockwise with their closed fist out in front of them clasped by their other hand. A more modern version involves taking a walk or run and paying attention to how your body feels when you move, becoming truly present, aware of the elements of nature evident on your journey. In shamanic practice, movement is thought to help release emotions we have supressed due to unresolved issues.

- **Mantra meditation**: this is an auditory technique. You can use a word, a phrase, a sound, a note or even a whole poem. Your word should be sacred to you and your intention in the meditation. A simple sound can be enough to focus the mind and quiet the chatter. You can chant, whisper or sound the words in your head. The pitch of certain notes will appear to resonate with you. You may want to sing one single note.

- **Loving kindness meditation**: this Buddhist technique is also called *metta* meditation. It adds intention to goodwill. It involves visualizing loved ones, feeling the love and kindness that they feel towards you and then sending it back to them. This technique was evaluated by Barbara Fredrickson.[1] She and her team showed long-lasting increases in positive thoughts. Further analysis showed a benefit to physical health and relationships.[2]

- **Shamanic meditations** (also known as **journeying**): this is one of the oldest forms of meditation (35,000 years). Altered states of awareness are achieved by drumming at a rate of 220 beats per minute, creating a specific frequency which evokes a trance state. With regular practice you can achieve a trance-like state without the need for the drumming. The purpose is to travel to hidden worlds to retrieve knowledge that will help us to affect positive change in our lives.

- **Body scan meditation**: the human body is a miraculous creation. It is filled with millions of sensory receptors which are constantly supplying us with masses of information. Most of this information does not make it into our conscious awareness, but the body does not need it to. We unconsciously respond all the time, making fine adjustments to stay healthy and maintain the status quo. Our bodies do this without our needing to think about it at all. How would it be if we really listened? A body scan meditation does just that – enabling us to focus on the sensations in our body, noting any areas of pain or vulnerability that need attention.
- **Transcendental meditation**: this technique is a specific silent mantra technique that is practised for 20 minutes, twice a day. It is taught by certified TM teachers using a copyrighted seven-step programme.

In all meditative techniques, it is possible to achieve true stillness with no thought at all. Deepak Chopra calls this 'slipping into the gap'.[3] Here is where we connect with the universe and have access to great wisdom.

The above list is far from exhaustive. Meditation is a fabulous skill to have, and it is easy to get started. Like any skill, it gets better with practice and perseverance.

Meditating on a particular issue

Meditation is often used as a relaxation exercise to clear the mind and bring us back into balance. It is possible, however, to meditate on a specific problem (e.g. resolving a dispute, achieving a goal or making an important decision). To do this, begin by setting a clear intention and be ready to receive. For example, 'I seek guidance about ...' The next step is to access the meditative state in one of the ways described above. When stillness is reached, 'slip into the gap' and await answers. Make sure you are listening and receptive to them.

Does it work?

Meditation has been the focus of much scientific study. It has been proven to have a beneficial effect on blood pressure, anxiety, depression, sleep, pain and cognitive function.[4] A recent systemic review of the evidence of its effect found meditation led to an increase in positive emotions and behaviours.[5] A more recent study showed that 15 minutes of meditation a day had a similar effect on mood and wellbeing as a day of holiday.[6]

Not all the research into meditation is positive. One recent study did demonstrate unpleasant sensations thought to be brought on by meditation.[7] However, this was more likely to be seen in subjects who already had high levels of negative thoughts. It is important to find a meditative practice that is right for you. If you experience unpleasant sensations, we would advocate observing that sensation without giving it emotional weight and analyse where it came from.

Practised regularly, meditation has the power to improve both our physical and psychological health. This is a core skill for building our resilience.

How to meditate

It is important to prepare your space as well as yourself for meditation. This sets a clear intention. Choose a time of day that suits you. Meditating in the morning can seem like an impossible feat, but setting your alarm and getting up early to meditate can make your day run more smoothly. In fact, you may feel as if you have gained time.

Some people meditate throughout the day to stay focused and reduce the stress and tension brought on by the workplace. Five minutes can be sufficient. Sometimes just refocusing your mind, letting go of all the current worries and stress, and allowing your body to relax is enough to get you back on track. Others use meditative exercises to help with sleep.

Whichever time you choose, make meditation a regular part of your day. Repetitive behaviours become habits, and this is one healthy habit. To make this a reality, add meditation on to an activity you already do every day. For example, you can get up, make the bed then sit down on the bed and meditate; or put the kettle on and, while you wait for it to boil, meditate. On the bus or train on the way to work you can listen to a guided meditation. When you get to work, switch on your computer and then, while you wait for it to boot up, you can take a few minutes to meditate. At lunchtime after you have eaten you can carve out 15 minutes for meditation. At home, after you have put the kids to bed and tidied up the general mess, and before you turn to the TV, you can take some time and meditate. Before you go to bed you can turn off all devices and give yourself the opportunity to go to bed with a calm and focused mind. If you wake at 3am worrying about something you forgot to do the day before or something looming in the future, you can use a meditation technique to tune those thoughts out and leave your mind calm and tranquil. Take the opportunities presented to you and make it work for you.

When you are ready to meditate

Whilst we advocate opportunistic meditation throughout the day, it is also beneficial to set aside dedicated time for this nourishing practice. This is about setting intention, honouring the Self and creating positive ritual.

1. Find a quiet place where you will not be disturbed. Prepare your space. Think about making it the perfect place for you to be. Think about the ambience. Is the light suitable? Is it warm and comfortable? Does the energy feel right? You can use essential oils to make it smell beautiful. The oils have different properties and can be used as part of the exercise. For example, lavender is thought to be calming, bergamot uplifting and frankincense balancing.

2. Prepare your body to meditate. Before you begin do a quick body-check. Are you hungry or thirsty? Do you need to go to the

toilet? Trying to meditate with a full bladder is difficult. Attend to your body before you begin.

3. Consider your posture. You need to be comfortable in order to meditate; you also need to be able to breathe fully and deeply, expanding your lungs. The ideal is sitting on a chair or the floor. If you are in a chair, make sure your bottom is to the back of the chair and your spine straight. You can lie down, though you may well fall asleep.

4. Prepare your mind to meditate. Set your intention. Are you aiming to relax and clear your mind? Are you meditating on a specific issue?

5. Take your awareness to your breathing. Feel your lungs expand and deflate. After a few deep breaths, start the meditative exercise you have chosen.

The most common problem people experience with meditation is distractions. External distractions will hopefully be taken care of by carefully preparing your space. Allow any little distractions, sounds or other pulls on your attention to become an accepted part of your experience. You can actually use them to drive you deeper into relaxation. To do this, set your intention by saying, 'Every sound I hear serves to make me even more relaxed.'

Internal distractions can be more difficult. These are the monkeys in your head demanding your attention. They will be many, and they will shout really loudly to get you to notice them. Calmly and gently bring your awareness back to your chosen focus. Imagine that you are speaking kindly and repetitively to a child. You will need to do this over and over again. This is normal – do not get discouraged. Just keep going. Over time, you will be able to achieve your focus more and more easily and hold it for longer periods of time.

Enjoy this beautiful core skill – it will serve you well. Have a look in Part 3 for many guided meditations with specific purposes.

13

Being present with mindfulness

Do not dwell in the past, do not dream of the future, concentrate your mind on the present moment.

The Buddha

We are constantly being told to be more mindful, but how do we do that? This chapter explains what mindfulness is, the reasons we need it, the value of it and what it can do for us. In Part 3 there is a fabulous tool called the White Room to help you achieve mindfulness.

Much is talked about mindfulness, being mindful and doing things mindfully. Do you know what it means? How it feels? Even if you have made some space in your life to practise mindfulness, how do you know if you have achieved it?

Jon Kabat-Zinn, the American professor who developed the mindfulness-based stress reduction (MBSR) programme, describes mindfulness as '*awareness* that arises through paying attention, on purpose, in the present moment, non-judgementally'.[1]

Eckhart Tolle calls mindfulness 'presence' and describes the state of presence as 'awareness without thought.'[2]

Mindfulness is about existing *in* the now, rather than through the filter of our thoughts *about* it.

A lot of the time our minds are full of thoughts; thoughts about the past and worries about the future. These include fears, remorse, guilt, shame and self-accusation, occasionally successes and happy memories, too. Most psychologists agree that the greater part of our thinking is repetitive. In fact, research suggests that 95 per cent of it is. Of this, 80 per cent is reported to be negative.[3] Let's remember that our thoughts affect body chemistry. We do not need to simulate past or future negative chemistry. When we come into the present moment, our needs are usually fairly basic. It is not often that we are actually experiencing negativity, however, when we are not present, we are regularly thinking about it.

Mindfulness is about being aware of all of our thoughts, but not being consumed by them. This means not attaching emotional weight to them. We can see our thoughts more clearly when we free ourselves from these attachments. When we truly observe our thoughts, watching them come and go, we become aware of patterns that signpost us to our conditioning, core beliefs, shadow and archetypes. Once we are aware of this information, we can act upon it.

The present moment also allows us to better connect to our unconscious mind. We become fully conscious and present in the situation. This enables us to channel information from the universe. We have both experienced this when talking to patients; times when we have been so present that exactly the right information and action has presented itself, without thought. Becoming in tune with the universe to affect healing is called *holding space*.[4] Being mindful is a core skill that allows us to do this for ourselves.

When we cultivate the habit of living mindfully, we become immersed in current tasks. Giving 100 per cent of our attention increases productivity, efficiency, attention to detail, compassion, retention of information, focus, creativity and execution of skill.

When we practise mindfulness, we can apply the core skill of observation and choice – Chapter 8.

Applications of mindfulness

There are many useful practical applications of mindfulness techniques:

- **Breaking bad habits**: eating when not fully present can lead to overconsumption.
- **Sleep**: when fully present, the mind cannot torture us with thoughts of past or future events and sleep habits improve.
- **Stress**: when fully present, we are only required to address any issue that is in the *now* so the mind cannot ruminate about numbers of problems.
- **Processing events, however traumatic**: situations which have created certain emotions can be broken down by consciously bringing them into the present moment. 'Sitting with' those emotions allows them to shift rather than pushing them away.
- **Addressing pain**: pain in the present moment requires either action or surrender. Accepting these as the only choices helps us to process it.
- **Reframing**: observing and recognizing when our thought patterns in the present are negative allows us to choose whether or not to reframe them. Reframing is discussed fully in Chapter 9.
- **Solitude**: in the modern world, we are facing increasing degrees of isolation. Mindfulness allows us to explore the serenity of silence brought about by freedom from the internal noise of our own thoughts.
- **Facing uncertainty**: again, the two choices in the present are action or surrender; appreciating this allows us to choose which and achieve peace.

Does mindfulness work?

There is extensive research into the effects of mindfulness. Investigations into the psychological effects of mindfulness have revealed that it brings about various positive psychological effects, including increased subjective wellbeing, reduced psychological symptoms and emotional reactivity, and improved behavioural regulation.[5] Further studies found strong, consistent evidence for benefits to cognitive and emotional reactivity, moderate and consistent evidence for mindfulness, rumination and worry, and preliminary but insufficient evidence for self-compassion and psychological flexibility.[6] Additionally, research has shown a positive relation between mindfulness and healthier eating.[7]

As with meditation, there is some research that questions the benefits. This, however, is very limited, and the main criticism is that it is difficult to undertake research in this field.

How to achieve mindfulness

- **Mindful activities:** pay attention to one thing instead of multitasking. Fully engage in the activity, activate all your senses, taking in all the sights, sounds and sensations it generates.
- **Mindful listening:** when speaking to someone, stop what you are doing and give them your full attention. This is mindful listening. Cultivate your stillness so that you do not let negative thoughts or emotions in your head get in the way of listening. Give people time to speak before jumping in. Pause before you reply and use that stillness to choose the right words.
- **Mindful meditation:** this is a great way to enjoy being present. This is described fully in Chapter 14. The first tool in Part 3 is a guided meditation to help you achieve mindfulness. It was created by Chrissie, who uses it with her patients on a daily basis. The White Room, as she calls it, gives you a visual anchor to the present moment. You can physically clear your White Room of thoughts and emotions. You can use your White Room whenever you need it, to process past events, reframe core beliefs and set positive intentions for the future. Dedicate time for mindful meditation and you will soon see the rewards. You can download and listen to the White Room for free by adding your email to our website <www.resilientpractice.co.uk>.

- **Mindful eating:** this involves paying attention to all of our senses. How the food looks, smells, tastes, the sounds made in the preparation, its texture. How your stomach feels when hungry and then when satisfied. Being present in your body allows you to get a fuller experience from meals and you will find that you eat less.[8]
- **Mindful colouring and drawing:** these are wonderfully creative ways to be mindful. Notice the patterns and colours. Be aware of the pencil on the paper.
- **Mindful moving:** this gives you the opportunity to become aware of your whole body in motion. If you are moving to music, be aware of how the rhythm feels in your body and how the music sounds to you. Observe the effect on your breathing and the feelings in your arms and legs. Note the heat generated by the movement and relax any tension you feel in your body. Walking mindfully allows us to connect to the immense power of the natural world.

Allowing mindfulness to become habitual in your life will bring peace and connection. Notice things around you and be curious. Be aware of the sensations in your body using all your senses: sight, hearing, smell, taste, touch. Be aware of your actions. Do not allow the awareness to generate thoughts that take you away from the present moment.

14

Harnessing rituals

When tea becomes ritual, it takes place at the heart of our ability to see greatness in small things.

Muriel Barbery

Ritual *(noun)*: A series of actions that are always performed in the same way, especially as part of a religious ceremony.

In this chapter, we discuss the presence of ritual across all cultures and its importance in human experience. We will discuss where ritual currently exists in our lives and how it serves us. Our rituals are the things we do over and over again. Human beings relish routine – it makes us feel safe and keeps us on track. We can learn to harness the power that resides within our rituals.

Rituals allow us to create time in which to celebrate, honour, cherish, give thanks, value, love, acknowledge, pledge, dedicate and grieve.

Our lives are full of rituals – from brushing our teeth, to the route we take to work, to the greetings we share with colleagues, to our work timetable, to our bedtime ritual; from the celebrations we attend to the rites of passage we go through. Many we call habits, but there is an important distinction. Habits tend to be unconscious; we just do them. The meaning we give to our rituals makes them conscious and brings them and us into the present moment.

The human practice of imbuing symbolic meaning in our chosen repetitive activities is what creates ritual. Rituals are present in all cultures. They are often associated with religion and spirituality but, in fact, rituals are threaded throughout our lives. They keep us safe (mirror–signal–manoeuvre), present (standard operating procedures) and connected (rites of passage). Our rituals are our structure and support. We recognize them, and with that recognition comes comfort.

Turning things on or off in the same order means that no item is missed. In medicine, consultation models are rituals that ensure healthcare professionals ask all the right questions, collecting every piece of relevant information and considering every possibility. They promote patient safety. Protocols or standard operating procedures (SOP) are present in many occupations. They remind us of how to do things, and they regulate our practice.

Rituals can be used to reduce anxiety. The familiarity of a recognized practice gives a sense of control, which improves our confidence.

Rituals welcome people into a community. They are the backbone for developing our social relationships. Sharing a ceremony connects us with our culture, with our family and friends, and with the wider community. Rituals honour our ancestors, allowing us to tap into their wisdom. We, in turn, are able to pass our wisdom on in the same way.

We mark the milestones in our life with rites of passage from birth through to our death. Honouring ourselves and others in this way ensures that these events do not pass by unnoticed. We also mark the changing of the seasons, asking for blessings for the new crops and giving thanks for the harvest.

Rituals help us to process grief. In a recent study, participants subjectively rated grief rituals as 'moderately to very helpful' in coping with loss.[1]

Some cultures use specific rituals to connect to the universe and receive abundance. Examples are: the Catholic Holy Communion, the Native American rain dance, the Japanese tea ceremony and fertility ceremonies performed across the globe. Rituals are extensively used as a tool for healing.

Performers of all spheres harness ritual to enhance their performance: musicians, actors, public speakers and those participating in sports. The pre-performance rituals that we attend to calm the mind. They are a way of focusing attention, bringing the performer into the present moment where anxiety about the upcoming performance has no place. The rituals are part of their mental preparation. Marcus Mumford (of the band Mumford & Sons) burns a stick of palo santo to clear his head. Rihanna prays, and Leonard Cohen had his band recite a Latin phase, 'Pauper sum ego, nihil habeo' ('I am poor, I have nothing').[2] Rafael Nadal has a specific pre-game ritual. While on the court, he ritualistically towels himself after every point, and he will not stand up to restart play before his opponent.[3] Tiger Woods always wears a red top for Sunday matches. His mother says, 'It is his power colour.'

Sometimes our rituals come in the form of a superstition or good-luck charm. Karen had a Whitby duck that she took into every examination. Chrissie burns sage to cleanse her space before meditation. Rituals can be simple but are sacred to the Self.

Research

There is a significant body of research into rituals. Family routines and rituals have been associated with many benefits: higher marital satisfaction, adolescents' sense of personal identity, children's health, academic achievement and stronger family relationships.[4]

Rituals reduce anxiety, lower heart rate and improve performance, provided they are imbued with symbolic meaning. The improved performance was explained by a reduction in self-reported anxiety.[5]

Though rituals might appear, on the surface, to be wasteful in terms of time and energy expenditure, their presence in different performance contexts suggests they are critical to self-regulation and goal attainment.[6] Activating good-luck-related superstitions has been shown to improve performance in golfing, motor dexterity, memory, and anagram games through boosting participants' confidence, which, in turn, improved performance.[7] A study of adolescents compared two groups. The intervention group had been told that the symbol at the top of the test paper might bring them luck; the other group had no information about the symbols. The results showed that girls in the intervention group did better. This is thought to be by improving their belief in their ability to do well.[8]

It is clear that we must make the habits in our life conscious in order to harness their power. When they are conscious, we can assess whether or not they truly serve us, and, if they do not, we can choose to replace them with ones that do.

However, being overly attached to rituals, relying on them to stay afloat, can stop us from moving forward. When they are used to excess, we become stuck. We must apply the core skill of observation and choice, acknowledge the fear that is keeping us attached, and consciously decide to whether to let the pattern of behaviour run or not.

For example, the family gatherings associated with significant holidays will have multiple rituals woven deeply into them. We have all had the experience of slipping back into our old role in the family, even though we have moved forward in the rest of our lives. We do this sometimes, even to the point of reliving old disagreements. If these rituals bring up old hurts, we are masochistically repeating the same negative pattern. If we become conscious of the rituals in our lives, we can choose how to participate in any ritual and, therefore, harness its power rather than be consumed by it.

When our rituals do serve us, we can increase their power by imbuing them with meaning and purpose. This means we must set clear intentions. We must use our rituals to bring us into the present moment with a calm, focused mind. We must allow them to help us to rise.

Part 3 contains many tools that can become healthy rituals.

15

Keeping therapeutic records

I can shake off everything as I write; my sorrows disappear, my courage is reborn.

Anne Frank

In this chapter, we will consider how we process and record information, explaining the value of keeping therapeutic records. We will explore ways of recording events, thoughts, feelings and behaviours, thereby allowing us to process them. The way we choose to do this recording and processing will be very individual and may take many forms. Keeping records is not just about writing. We can use music, art and movement for self-expression, allowing us to sit with thoughts and feelings and then shift them. Examples include poetry, creative writing, dancing, sports, sculpture, crafts, singing, chanting and turning up the music.

Learning styles

Before we consider therapeutic records, it is important we understand the way we learn. This is a vast and extremely interesting subject. For the purposes of this book, we want to share some key theories to help you understand how we best process knowledge, as this is the way we move forwards. This will also help you to choose resilience tools and understand why you like some things and not others. Choosing tools that resonate with you will improve their effectiveness.

In the 1990s, Peter Honey and Alan Mumford described four different learning styles. They identified the Activist, the Pragmatist, the Reflector and the Theorist.[1]

The Activist learns best by doing. The Pragmatist learns via practical demonstrations. The Reflector learns by watching and then thinking about what they have seen. The Theorist needs to understand the theory underlying the concept. Part 3 is a toolbox of exercises and techniques from which you can build your own Resilience Toolkit. Reflectors will like the journalling exercises. Theorists will be attracted to the techniques with a solid theoretical basis. Pragmatists will love the practical strategies and guided meditations. The Activists will dive in and try exercises that involve action.

While these theories of learning styles are useful, it is very important that we do not allow ourselves to be constrained by them. In fact, there has been research to suggest that we learn best by using all four modalities. We would encourage you to give all the tools a go, thinking about what you want to achieve. Use the right tool for the job!

The next model to discuss is the VAK model of learning modalities.[2] This model was briefly touched on in Chapter 11. Barbe and his team described three ways of learning and hypothesized that everyone has a modality through which they learn the best. Interestingly, this may not be their preferred way of learning. The three modalities are visual, auditory and kinaesthetic. Visual learners respond best to material they can see, such as pictures and diagrams. Auditory learners like to listen and take part in discussions. Kinaesthetic learners like to use movement in a hands-on way.

As we mentioned in Chapter 11, Chrissie is an auditory learner. She loves listening to audiobooks. Karen is more kinaesthetic but actually has elements of all three.

Critics of this model state that assigning a learning modality is too rigid and can encourage a narrow approach to learning. When we accept labels, we are constrained by them. In truth, there is no ideal. We all learn in different ways – the key is to recognize our own learning style and preferences so we choose learning activities to suit. Once again, this is the core skill observation and choice (Chapter 8). We should also consider expanding our learning style by trying other modalities. The most flexible learners are comfortable with all three.[3]

Our toolbox contains tools that cover all three modalities and, where possible, we have given VAK options. We wholeheartedly urge you to embrace all three.

We have discussed learning styles, and you will now have an idea of your own strengths and preferences. Now we will discuss how to apply these in keeping therapeutic records.

Why we keep records

Safeguarding and improving our practice

In the medical world, when something goes wrong we take a detailed look at what happened so all involved can learn from the event, in the hope that systems and processes can be strengthened to make sure that it does not happen again. We call this *significant event analysis* (SEA). In a similar way, keeping a therapeutic record of our day – things that have gone well, things that have not gone so well and what could have been done differently – will help you process the events. This is not about blame; it is about taking all the lessons from our lives and using them to help us and others to *rise*.

Identifying and reframing thoughts and core beliefs

Thought diaries have been used in cognitive behavioural therapy (CBT) for years. There are many types, but the principle is the same. Write down your thoughts and feelings and then try to note where there are cognitive illusions.[4] This is where our thoughts are distorted by our emotions. We do this when we have something to gain from it – for example catastrophizing, jumping to conclusions, making assumptions, fortune telling, mind reading, selective evidence gathering and overgeneralizing. Unhelpful thinking patterns, once identified, can then be challenged. We would recommend that readers take a step further and use their thought record to identify core beliefs. Negative core beliefs can then be reframed.

The thought diary below is specifically designed to allow you to pick out repetitive thought patterns, which, in turn, will allow you to identify associated core beliefs. Challenging our thoughts without reframing the underlying core beliefs will not fully address the issue.

Date	Event	Thoughts and feelings	Cognitive illusions and distorted thinking	Core belief	Reframe

When we evaluate our thoughts and core beliefs we must *detach* from any associated emotions. Again, this is the core skill observation and choice. We can then analyse the evidence for and against those thoughts and beliefs in a calm, methodical manner. We can then reframe them to suit us.

For example, a common negative thinking pattern consists of 'I am so stupid. Why did I do that?' The core belief underlying this thinking is 'I am stupid.'

'My brother always gets to go first ... This must mean my parents love him more than me ... This must mean I am not loveable.' The underlying core belief here is 'I am unlovable.'

'John got a pay rise and I didn't ... This means I am not as good at the job as John ... This means I am no good.' The underlying core belief is 'I am worthless.'

Let us analyse the first example. Detaching and evaluating without feelings of guilt and shame we can ask: 'Is this true?'

'Do I mean "stupid" or do I mean "unprepared"?' 'In fact, did I have the required information to perform the task?'

Reframe the original thought using the following observations: 'Things did not go as I hoped today. I did not perform the task correctly ... I did not have the appropriate amount of knowledge,' and change to 'I have learned that I need to be better prepared.' Prepare, and then set the intention: 'Tomorrow I will go back and perform my task well.'

The reframed core belief is thus: 'I am intelligent and capable.'

Part 3 contains several reframing tools.

Record-keeping for expression and release

The physical act of keeping therapeutic records is a way of expressing and processing everything that has happened to us in our day. Creative writing, dance, music and art are all expressive forms of therapeutic record-keeping. Using these methods of recording is just as valuable as writing things down formally. Consider the benefits of recording in a conscious way. How we choose to catalogue our day is entirely personal. A particularly visual person may be drawn to using photographs or drawings or paintings. An auditory person, to music – either playing or listening. A more kinaesthetic person may want to reflect on their day by creating something – a sculpture, a meal or by dancing out their feelings.

Does keeping therapeutic records work?

There is a plethora of literature detailing the benefits of keeping therapeutic records to express and process our day, for mind body and spirit. Creative writing was found to reduce intrusive and avoidant thinking about a stressful experience.[5] It has been shown to reduce blood pressure.[6] After some short-term negative symptoms, subjects showed improvements in multiple self-reported symptoms and objective measures.[7] The team found fewer stress-related visits to the doctor, improved immune system functioning, reduced blood pressure, improved lung function, improved liver function, fewer days in hospital, improved mood/affect, fewer post-traumatic and avoidance symptoms, and increased feelings of psychological wellbeing. The authors concluded that the most likely explanation for the results was that the writing allowed cognitive processing of events. A more recent study evaluating an online 'positive affect journalling' programme found that it was an effective intervention for alleviating mental distress, increasing wellbeing, and enhancing physical functioning.[8] A review of over 800 studies showed that dance movement therapy is an effective intervention in the treatment of adults with depression.[9] The same has been found in music, with a review of 28 studies showing a statistically significant reduction in depression levels over time.[10] Similarly with art, data collected from more than 23,000 participants showed that arts engagement among the population as a whole may help enhance positive mental health and life satisfaction, protecting against mental distress.[11]

In practice, we have found many additional benefits to keeping therapeutic records, including that the confidential nature of our record means that we can express whatever we need to, as there is no audience. The convenience of having our own record means we can do it when it suits us. It helps us to organize our thoughts and it can serve as a record of our progress.

Therapeutic records allow us to be accountable for what has happened in our lives. Part 3 contains tools that utilize various types of therapeutic record-keeping.

16

Creating a resilient mind-set

> Everything can be taken from a man but one thing: the last
> of the human freedoms – to choose one's attitude in any
> given set of circumstances, to choose one's own way.
>
> *Viktor E. Frankl*

Mind-set *(noun)*: A set of attitudes or fixed ideas that someone
has and that are often difficult to change.

Attitude *(noun)*: The way that you think and feel about
somebody/something; the way that you behave towards
somebody/something that shows how you think and feel.

We would like to challenge the first definition. It is entirely
possible and, in fact, imperative that we learn how to change
our mind-set. This is vital in moving forward and overcoming
inertia.

Have you ever had someone described to you as having 'a
sunny disposition'? Did you look for the sunshine in that person
when you met them or was it evident in their outlook? Did you
wonder how they got to see the world in such a positive light?

In this chapter, we are going to show you how to observe
your own mind-set and choose to shape it according to how you
want to see the world.

We have discussed, at great length, how, along with our
genetic make-up, our unique set of experiences has shaped
our model of the world. This is the lens through which we
see everything. It matches the core beliefs that arise from it. It
therefore colours our thoughts, emotions and behaviours. These

behaviours become our responses and reactions when we are provoked by the external environment.

Throughout life, the cycle of core beliefs, thoughts, emotions and responses becomes repetitive. When we are not self-aware, we are not even conscious of these repetitive patterns; to us they are the norm. This habitual way of thinking, feeling and responding becomes our *mind-set*. As we have discussed throughout this book, core beliefs and thoughts can be reframed. If we can reframe these, then we can shape our mind-set. Cultivating a resilient mind-set will result in positive, repetitive patterns of thinking and behaviour. Imagine how this would benefit all aspects of life.

To do this we are, once again, required to observe and choose. We are also required to overcome resistance. We discussed overcoming resistance in detail in Chapter 6, when we looked at survival archetypes. When we walk towards something in life, we are always walking away from something else. Identifying what we are unconsciously walking towards is the first step in shaping our mind-set. We can use our powers of self-awareness to do this.

By choosing to walk towards one thing and away from another, we are activating universal laws. By walking towards something we give it our *attention*. The mind-set we choose determines what we *attract* into our life. These are the universal laws discussed in detail in Chapter 4.

To achieve a resilient mind-set, we need to consciously walk in the following directions:

- from indifference towards gratitude
- from empathy towards compassion
- from resistance towards acceptance/surrender
- from external towards internal (locus of control)
- from illness towards health (including mental health)
- from fear towards love.

Walking from indifference towards gratitude

When we accept gains without expressing gratitude, we are indifferent. When we are indifferent, we lose the opportunity to accentuate the gain. According to the Universal Law of Attraction, we will receive indifference rather than abundance. In choosing to be grateful, we align our energy to universal abundance. When we consider ourselves to be fortunate, we believe that we have abundance and therefore the universe reflects that abundance.

Let's now examine the things for which we can be grateful. During our workshops, we ask people to write down what they are grateful for. Often, they have to think about this before writing. If we have to look for things to be grateful for, we are not living gratefully. A grateful mind-set would not require us to look. We would automatically see the gift in every single moment, regardless of whether it was pleasant or not.

There are the obvious things that you can pick out as positive, for example a compliment or a pay rise, a gift, someone holding the door for you, a meal you enjoyed. When fostering gratitude, it is easy to acknowledge these. It is also traditional to list all the things in our lives we are grateful for, such as our family, friends, work and possessions. This is where most people stop. The problem with stopping here is that, in order to feel grateful, we *need* these nice things in our lives. These things are, in fact, attachments. This means that anything that affects them also affects us. This externalizes our locus of control.

In addition to those obvious things for which we are grateful, all moments of adversity contain gifts. When we experience hardship, we must foster gratitude for the lessons we have learned. This is not easy but it is living gratefully, and living gratefully attracts abundance. For example, when we lose someone we love, we can choose to be grateful because the sorrow we feel is a product of the joy that we experienced with that person.

We have described how to be grateful when events are good and when they are terrible. What about everything in between? How do we live gratefully in our daily grind? We do this by recognizing all our gains and what brought them to us. For example, when you are swamped with work, be grateful for the opportunity to serve. Remember that you asked for that opportunity and it was granted. When you are driven insane by the school run, in addition to being grateful for your beautiful children, be grateful for the lesson given to you. It's a lesson in the value of better organization and setting off on time!

True resilience is living gratefully. Living gratefully involves not only counting our blessings but acknowledging that *every moment* is a blessing.

Walking from empathy towards compassion

In the modern world, empathy is widely extolled as a virtue. We are praised when we demonstrate it. We are taught it in medical school. We would like to explore empathy in more detail so you can be mindful of its effect upon you and the people with whom you empathize. Empathy arises in our interactions – we are either the empath or the recipient of empathy.

Empathizing with others

When we empathize, we tell ourselves that we are actually feeling the emotions of another person. These can be positive or negative. It is not possible to feel someone else's emotions, only our own.

Given that everything is subject to the Universal Law of Reflection, the version of the person we see is created by us. Remember, we never really know a person fully; we only know the version of them that we have created based on our model of the world. What we are we feeling is projection. We project in two ways: how we would feel in their situation, or how we think our version of them would feel. We also project our own need to be perceived as caring.

Projection is always expressed either verbally or non-verbally. It therefore always impacts on the other person. The effect of this is to pull the locus of power away from them. For example, people with a cancer diagnosis can be reluctant to share the news because they are unconsciously aware that negative emotions will be projected upon them. This can impact on their power to heal.

When someone excitedly tells us about a new project, in empathizing we can project our own self-doubt upon them and deny them the ability to achieve. Parents often do this with comments like 'Don't take on too much' and 'Don't get your hopes up.' They do this to protect us. They are actually projecting their own fear of failure.

Why do we do this? What we project arises from our core beliefs, so empathizing gives us the opportunity to affirm them. Affirmation of negative core beliefs drives the cognitive behavioural cycle, stimulating release of the negative body chemicals that we crave. When we are empathizing we are *always* projecting. Making assumptions about how others are feeling is an imposition and not consensual. It will always have consequences.

Being the recipient of empathy

Quite often, we find ourselves sharing bad news more widely than we need. What do we get from this? Accepting empathy legitimizes our negative cognitive behavioural cycles. We recruit allies who project negative emotions on to us, giving us permission to perpetuate our own. Why do we share our achievements? Sometimes it's to reaffirm our delicate positive core beliefs, but, often, we are trying to convince ourselves through others that we are good enough. In order to avoid attracting empathy from others we need to examine why we are seeking a response. We may be asking for approval, affirmation of worth, validation of our emotions or nurture. We can provide these for ourselves. We do not need to seek an external response. In providing these things for ourselves and allowing others to do the same, we are walking towards compassion; for ourselves and others.

Compassion

We would like to suggest that compassion is a more resilient response to the request for empathy. When we are invited to empathize, we can use the core skill observation and choice. We observe our immediate reactions and explore where they come from. We can then consciously choose compassion over empathy.

As explained above, when we give empathy, our own emotions contaminate the situation. When we are compassionate, we put our emotions on hold. We actively listen to the needs of the other person and, rather than reacting because of how we feel, we consciously respond with respect. We offer our services and expertise with intelligence, understanding and kindness. We have learned that offering help and advice to people who have not asked for it can be harmful to both parties and the relationship. It interrupts their progress and comes from our need to help. When feedback is asked of us, it is imperative that we step back from our emotions. This requires detachment. There are tools for detaching in Part 3.

Walking from resistance towards acceptance

We have talked a great deal about resistance to our progress in Chapters 6 and 8. When we resist our current circumstances, we deny ourselves a state of acceptance. Living in a state of acceptance is an essential requirement for creating a resilient mind-set. We need to accept hardship, abundance and uncertainty.

Accepting hardship

When terrible things happen, we are at a loss to accept them. These are the most challenging times of our lives. Much of our energy is taken up in resisting what has happened. This creates, within us, a black hole which constantly drains our energy. The most resilient course of action is to change what we can change and accept what remains. We cannot change past events. We can acknowledge how terrible the situation is but, when we rage against the machine, we are powerless. It is like pushing really hard against a brick wall which will not move. This is why grief can feel exhausting. Walking towards acceptance during hardship is an extremely difficult journey. It is, however, the only way to eventually move forward.

Accepting abundance

Accepting abundance means that, when we are presented with gifts, we must be open to receiving them. Such gifts might be, love, friendship, possessions and compliments. When these things are offered to us, we sometimes find ourselves pushing them away. This is resistance. It comes from a place of fear. This fear arises when we feel we are not worthy or good enough to receive such gifts. These are negative core beliefs. In order to accept abundance, we must observe those responses within us and choose to reframe them. Chapters 9 and 14 go into detail about reframing. There are also tools to address this in Part 3.

Accepting uncertainty

It is impossible to go through life without experiencing uncertainty. Uncertainty generates fear. In accepting uncertainty, we conserve our energy. We have talked a great deal about our threat responses. What if, when something happens to us that is beyond our control, we see it is an opportunity to address how we might survive? What if we see it as an invitation?

In fact, uncertainty is an opportunity to learn about the Self and to develop tools for self-preservation.

- Start by coming into the present moment. The only thing that matters is what is happening right now.
- What do you feel right now?
- What are your current needs? Are they pretty basic? Oxygen? Shelter? Nourishment? Comfort?
- Is there anything that poses a problem right now?
- You can either do something about it or accept it. Those are the only choices.
- Take any action that you can and accept what remains.

Accepting everything is a key part of the core skill of creating a resilient mind-set. Buddhists believe that nothing stays the same. This belief can help us through times of transition and pain. In acceptance we know that whatever we must endure will change. Acceptance is a beautiful thing.

Walking from an external to an internal locus of control

As discussed in Chapter 1, our locus of control is the extent to which we believe we have the power to affect change in our lives. The locus of control is a spectrum and we all sit at some point along it. Where we sit can also change depending on our current circumstances. Those whose locus of control is more external are more likely to say, and indeed believe, things like: 'There is nothing I can do about it', 'It's not what you know, it's who you know' and 'Life is down to luck. It doesn't matter what I do.'

Such people often feel powerless or victimized. They blame others for what happens and how they feel, and they seek approval from others. To have an external locus of control is to tell yourself that you are powerless; you have no control over what happens in your life. Giving away responsibility for our thoughts and feelings disempowers us and leaves us vulnerable and without resilience.

In contrast, those with a strong internal locus of control say and believe things like: 'It's up to me', 'I control my own destiny', 'If I work hard, I will achieve' and 'You make your own luck.' They think in an optimistic way. They actively look for solutions to problems. They are happier, healthier and more resilient.

Our position on the spectrum is not fixed. In fact, we can choose to walk towards the internal end of the spectrum, if we want to. We do this by being aware of what we can and cannot control. Factors we cannot control are our limitations, and energy spent trying to change them is wasted. We acknowledge that we are fully in control of all of our thoughts, feelings and behaviours. No one has the power to affect our emotions unless we choose to let them.

We can reframe negative responses. When we notice a negative response in ourselves, this may be physical – a sick feeling in our stomach, a tight chest or palpitations; or a thought – I'm not good enough, I have failed. We can stop and take a moment to examine that response. We can ask ourselves:

- Why has this response been triggered?
- Is my response appropriate?
- Is my response helpful?
- Is there a different response that would be more appropriate, more useful?

In walking towards an internal locus of control, we are taking responsibility for all our responses.

Walking away from illness towards health (including mental health)

When we have a mind-set for good health, we activate the Universal Law of Attraction. This means we will attract wellness.

Walking towards an attitude of good health is vital for creating a resilient mind-set. This may seem like an obvious statement. Why would anyone ever walk towards illness? We can explore this question by asking, 'What do I have to lose by being well?'

In truth, we are all attached to our pain to some degree. This is because we have perceived it to be part of us. There are many reasons why people walk towards illness – for example the loving care they receive from others, financial benefits, shedding responsibility and being the centre of attention. You will recognize elements of the survival archetypes in these examples. These are obstacles to moving forward. If we want to walk towards health, we must be brave. We must ask ourselves to observe our emotional relationship with our pain. Where might any of these obstacles be at play?

Here you can use the core skill of observation and choice. Identify and acknowledge what is happening and choose whether or not to allow it. *Evolve or repeat.*

Walking away from fear towards love

Everything we have discussed so far allows us to consciously choose to walk away from what does not serve us, towards what nourishes us. This is walking away from *fear* towards *love*. Creating a resilient mind-set activates the Universe Law of Attraction. It allows us to thrive in the present moment, whatever is happening. It enables us to move forward in a positive way.

17

What next?

Now, Voyager, sail thou forth, to seek and find.

Walt Whitman

We have given you everything you need for your journey of
    self-discovery.

You know the destination.

You understand the waters.

Your vessel is prepared and ready.

We have shown you the map.

All you need are the tools for your journey.

Part 3 is a comprehensive toolbox.

Come aboard and build your own Resilience Toolkit.

You will now stay afloat, whatever the weather.

Enjoy the voyage!

Part 3
THE RESILIENCE TOOLBOX

18

Introduction to the toolbox

I have a thing for tools!

Tim Allen

Here is your resilience toolbox. It consists of 60 of our favourite tools from which you can make your own, individual Resilience Toolkit. They are organized into three sections: meditations with purpose, guided visualizations and practical exercises.

To help you find the right tool for the job we have devised a key. In the table below is a list of common problems. Each problem has a specific set of tools mapped to it. These are the most effective for that situation.

The second table contains 'The Resilience Gap Analysis' questions from Chapter 1. Remember that these cover important aspects of resilience and highlight where you are most in need of resilience tools. Again, the most appropriate tools have been mapped.

Each tool has an indication of which problems and resilience questions it will help you with. This means that you can either begin with a problem or by exploring the toolbox itself.

We have been very specific with the key to make it prescriptive, but do not allow this to limit you. All the meditations will relax you, many of the exercises will bring you into the present, and relaxation and mindfulness help with many conditions.

There are eight *Super Tools* which are universal and can be used to move forward positively, in any situation. Rather than include them in the key we have listed them here for your attention. We recommend that you familiarize yourself with them. They will form the backbone of your Resilience Toolkit. In the absence of a type of tool in either key, look to these.

- **M4 Breathing meditation**
- **M11 Gratitude meditation**
- **M17 The White Room mindfulness meditation**
- **V2 Balancing visualization**
- **V12 Ideal future visualization**
- **P6 Five-point rescue plan**
- **P7 Gratitude journal**
- **P22 Thought reframe**

Key	Specific problem	Appropriate tools
A	Anxiety	M3 M6 M12 M13 M14 M18 M19 M21 V1 V3 V4 V6 V8 V9 V11 V13 V14 V16 P1 P2 P10 P16 P18 P19 P20 P23
B	Depression	M2 M12 M13 M14 M18 M19 M20 M21 V1 V4 V6 V8 V10 V11 V15 P2 P10 P11 P18 P19 P20
C	Stress	M3 M6 M8 M12 M13 M14 V1 V4 V8 V9 V11 V14 V15 P2 P3 P10 P14 P17 P18 P20 P21
D	Low self-worth	M1 M2 M5 M7 M8 M10 M13 M15 M16 V5 V6 V8 V10 V11 P1 P4 P9 P10 P11 P12 P15 P16 P19 P20
E	Panic attack	M6 M12 M18 V4 V9 V13 V14 P12 P16 P23
F	Trauma	M2 M5 M7 M9 M10 M13 M16 M18 M21 V1 V4 V5 V6 V8 V13 P2 P23
G	Adverse conditioning	M1 M2 M5 M7 M9 M10 M13 M15 M16 V6 P1 P8 P12 P15 P16 P19 P20
H	Loss	M1 M7 M8 M9 M10 M14 M16 M18 M20 V1 V5 V8 V11 V15 P2 P10
I	Insomnia	M3 V3 V9 V15 V16

J	Weight loss	M19 M21 V6 V7 P8 P11 P19
K	IBS	M3 M19 M21 V7 P19
L	Breaking habits	M5 M7 M9 M15 M16 V6 P8 P19
M	Addiction	M3 M5 M7 M9 M15 M16 V6 P8 P19
N	Relationship problems	M1 M2 M8 M18 V5 V6 V15 P1 P2 P3 P8 P9 P10 P12 P13 P17 P20
O	Improving performance	M9 V7 V10 V11 P2 P3 P4 P5 P9 P11 P12 P14 P17 P20 P21
P	Communication	M1 M8 P1 P3 P9 P10 P12 P13
Q	Reframing core beliefs	M5 M7 M9 M13 M15 M16 P4 P8 P15 P16 P19
R	Managing fear	M6 M7 M10 M12 M15 M16 M18 V1 V3 V8 V10 V11 V13 V14 V16 P4 P12 P16 P18 P19 P23
S	Pain	M2 M3 M10 M12 M13 M14 M19 M20 M21 V1 V4 V6 V7 V8 V9 V10 V13 V15 P2 P18
T	Isolation	M2 M20 V1 V7 V10 V11 P10 P13 P17 P18

	Gap analysis question	Appropriate tools
1	How well do you manage your workload?	M14 P1 P2 P3 P5 P8 P9 P14 P21
2	How well do you cope with uncertainty?	M6 M12 M14 V1 V8 V13 V14 P2 P4 P8 P16 P19 P20

3	How much of your time do you spend ruminating about past/future events?	M6 M7 M9 M10 M13 M15 M16 V3 V7 V13 V14 V16 P2 P4 P15 P16 P18 P19
4	How often do you find yourself absorbing the emotional distress felt by others?	M1 M3 M7 M8 M9 M13 M15 M16 V5 V6 V15 P8 P13 P17
5	How often do you go home feeling significantly drained of energy?	M3 M6 M8 M10 M13 M14 M19 M20 M21 V7 V9 V10 V11 V14 V15 P3 P9 P17 P18 P20

6	How much pressure do you put on yourself to achieve your goals?
	  a. Professional
	  b. Personal
		M5 M7 M9 M15 M16 M19 M21
		V7 V11
		P3 P4 P8 P15 P16 P19

7	How do you rate your health habits in terms of
	  a. Sleep?
	  b. Physical activity?
	  c. Diet?
		M3 M5 M6 M15 M19 M20 M21
		V3 V4 V6 V7 V9 V10 V15 V16
		P8 P11 P17 P18 P19 P20

8	How do you rate your work–life balance (e.g., working late or at home)?	M5 M6 M14 P1 P2 P3 P5 P8 P9 P14 P15 P17
9	How do you rate your organizational skills?	P2 P3 P5 P8 P9 P11 P14 P21
10	How well do you manage your time?	M6 P2 P3 P5 P8 P9 P11 P14 P21

11	How well do you communicate with
	  a. Family and friends?
	  b. Colleagues?
		M1 M8
		V5
		P1 P3 P10 P12 P13

12	How well do you manage inappropriate requests from
	  a. Family and friends?
	  b. Colleagues?
		M1 M5 M7 M8 M9 M15 M16
		V5 V6 V15
		P1 P9 P10 P12 P13 P14

13	How well do you process irritation caused by a. Family and friends? b. Colleagues?	M1 M2 M3 M8 M9 M14 M15 V4 V5 V6 V10 V15 P12 P17 P18 P19
14	How well do you adapt to change?	M10 M12 V10 V11 V13 P4 P16 P23
15	How well do you cope when things go wrong?	M6 M7 M12 M16 M18 V1 V8 V10 V11 V13 P2 P16 P17 P23
16	How well supported do you feel by your peers?	M1 M2 M10 M12 M19 M20 M21 V1 V5 V6 V8 V10 P1 P4 P10 P15 P17 P18
17	How supportive are your social relationships?	M1 M2 M10 M12 M19 M20 M21 V1 V5 V6 V8 V10 P1 P10 P15 P17 P18
18	How comfortable are you in sharing experiences with peers?	V5 V7 V10 V13 P1 P4 P10 P18 P20
19	How well do you process feedback?	M1 M2 M5 M7 M8 M9 M13 M15 M16 V1 V4 V6 V8 P1 P2 P12 P13 P15 P16 P19
20	How well do you manage conflict?	M1 M5 M6 M7 M8 M9 M12 M13 M14 M15 M18 M21 V1 V4 V8 V10 V11 V14 V15 P1 P2 P12 P13 P18 P19 P20 P23

19

Meditations with purpose

M1: Appreciating difficult relationships meditation

Specific issues	D G H N P
Gap analysis	4 11 12 13 16 17 19 20

It is undoubtedly good for us to be surrounded by people who love us, but what about the people who bring out the worst of our doubts and fears about our own self-worth and likeability? These relationships are important, too. They show us clearly where we need to work on our own personal growth. This meditative exercise helps us to gain the most from all of our relationships.

Use this tool after conflict with others, when someone has put you down, or difficult conversations within close personal relationships. Use it to gain closure and personal resolution, to invoke acceptance and peace.

Choose a moment where you are calm and centred and unlikely to be disturbed.

Bring your awareness to your breathing.

The tidal in and out of your breath.

This brings you into the present moment and allows you to focus.

Now bring to mind someone from the past or present with whom you have experienced difficulty connecting.

Someone who has never 'got' you.

Someone who has given you the impression that you were not 'liked'.

Maybe someone who has had the ability to make you feel small or unworthy.

These people easily spring to mind as they are the people who have hurt us.

Whether they know it or not.

Get a clear sense of that person.

Now examine how thinking of that person makes you feel.

How does it express itself in your body?

What thoughts spring to mind?

What fears come up for you?

Not good enough?

Not clever? Not beautiful?

Understand that none of this discord was about you for them.

Rather, it was all about what was going on for *them*.

The fact that you were triggered into unhappiness only displays a need within you.

For some kind of nurture that is separate from that person.

That person only served to show you the way.

You can provide that nurture.

How does that feel?

Can you *accept* the teaching?

Give yourself the gift of learning about your own needs from difficult relationships. Harbouring feelings of resentment towards those who have exposed our vulnerabilities serves only to hurt us further. When we do this, situations remain unresolved. What we leave unresolved keeps part of us forever in the past, and so we are blocked from moving forward.

If you can, offer a message of forgiveness and even gratitude to the people in your life who taught you the hardest lessons. Forgiveness does not signal approval of bad behaviour, but it does set us free, cutting any cords that bind us to people who dislike us. It helps us to detach.

Now picture someone who values you the highest of all.

Someone who loves you or respects you.

Without you having to do anything at all.

Maybe someone with whom you passionately share opinions.

Perhaps a partner.

Or a work colleague.

Or a friend.

Someone who appreciates your art, your song.

Your creativity.

Your beauty and your kindness.

Someone who really *sees* you.

Get a clear picture of that person.

How does that make you feel?

Where do you feel it in your body?

Remember that that person is evoking in you that which is *already there.*

Those are your emotions.

They do not belong to anybody else.

Sit with those pleasant feelings for a few minutes and allow yourself to be graced with gratitude. These are the relationships that we treasure.

By accepting all of our multifaceted relationships with others, we can begin to nurture and grow the most important relationship of all – our relationship to the Self.

M2: Authentic true self-meditation

Specific issues	B D F G N S T
Gap analysis	13 16 17 19

We were born with a set of genetic information and boundless potential. Everything else is a label or role we have accepted.

Use this tool to connect with the true authentic part of the Self, unaffected by your conditioning, and access that unbound potential.

Take your awareness to your breathing.

The tidal in and out of your breath.

As you do this, begin to allow that breath to slow and deepen.

Deeply and slowly.

Become aware of the feeling of calm that settles over you.

And now begin to allow the out breath to become just a little
bit longer than the in breath.

Picture the most authentic version of yourself.

Your true form.

What do you look like?

How does it feel to be you?

If you work, see yourself in your work role.

What qualities does that Self possess?

Why did you choose that role?

See yourself in your relationship.

Who are you as a partner?

What role do you play?

If you have children, see yourself as a parent.

How do you regard yourself as a parent?

Are you nurturing?

Are you firm with strong boundaries?

If you are a sibling, see yourself in that role.

What kind of brother or sister are you?

Which one are you?

The quiet one? The outgoing one? The clever one? The
creative one?

How would they describe you?

See yourself as a son or daughter.

How do you see yourself in this role?

What would they say about you?

Picture yourself in the centre of a large sphere.

Surrounding you are these roles that you have chosen to take
up.

With all their labels.

Their qualities and their descriptions.

Create some distance between yourself and them.

Understand that they are not you.

They are only roles that you have chosen to play.

They are not who you are.

The roles you have chosen in life are roles that have helped you to affirm the approved version of yourself.

Who approves?

Before you were recognized as being a certain sex.

You were someone.

Before you were seen someone's son or daughter.

You were someone.

Before you had a name.

You were someone.

Before you were understood to be a sibling.

You were someone.

Before you became someone's partner.

You were someone.

Before you chose your current roles.

You were someone.

Now take your awareness to your true authentic self.

Who are you?

Without the labels?

Own your whole multidimensional self with all of its darkness and light.

It is wonderfully complex. Embrace every aspect of that true being.

Approve of every facet of you.

Now give yourself permission to find your true essence.

Breathe it in.

Give it the gift of total acceptance.

And total approval.

And now gently let the images fade.

And bring yourself back to your current surroundings.

M3: Body scan meditation

Specific issues	A C I K M S
Gap analysis	4 5 7 13

This meditation helps us to connect with our body. Our body is our oldest and most loyal friend. The connection that this meditation affords us allows us to listen and respond to our body's needs. It also allows us to be grateful for the relationship.

Use this tool as part of your regular Self-care regimen.

Find a comfortable place to sit with your spine straight.

Take your awareness to your breathing.

The tidal in and out of your breath.

The rise and fall of your chest and abdomen.

Allow those breaths to slow and deepen and feel your body begin to relax and let go.

Let go of any tension that you have been holding within your muscles.

Tell your body to let it go.

Your body is *listening*.

As you sit completely still, what can you *feel*?

What information are you receiving?

Can you feel your breath? Your heartbeat? The weight of your body in the chair?

Sensation of your clothes against your skin?

Thank your body for the information and let it know that you are listening, too.

Now step into the shoes of your Observer Self and take a trip around your body.

Move steadily and gently through your head, neck, torso and limbs, noting all of the sensations that are felt.

Be aware of any area of the body where you feel pain or vulnerability.

Be aware of where you need to heal.

Thank your body for the information.

Know that, even when you seek help with healing, that healing comes from your body.

As you sit quietly, ask your body what obstacles there are to your healing.

What are your barriers? Your attachments?

Ask your body to help you to remove and release these now. Visualize them dissolving.

However you see this happening is right for you.

Feel a sense of freedom and liberation from that which has been holding you back.

Now give your body *permission* to heal.

Notice what happens as you do this.

Sit comfortably in the silence.

Spend a few minutes relaxing before you bring yourself back to full awareness with a new, profound love and appreciation for your body.

M4: Breathing meditation

SUPERTOOL

Specific issues	A–T
Gap analysis	1–20

Breathing is a core skill, and this is a universal meditation.

Use this technique on a daily basis as part of your wellbeing ritual. In addition, when you find yourself in a difficult situation, pause and use this tool to shift the negative energy. Then you can process what has happened in a positive frame of mind. In doing this, the outcome of the situation will be very different.

Sit in a comfortable position in a quiet space with your spine straight. Drop your shoulders and release any tension that you feel in your body.

Take your awareness to your breathing.

The tidal in and out of your breath.

Feel your 'aliveness'.

Now begin to allow your breath to slow and deepen.

Concentrate on allowing the out breath to become just a little bit longer than the in breath.

It is widely understood that, during the in breath, the tension in our muscles increases slightly and, during the out breath, our muscle tone decreases and allows us to 'let go'.

When thoughts outside the breathing arrive, just let them come and go without taking up space, and gently bring your awareness back to your breathing.

Now that you are calmly focused on your breathing:

Begin to see the in breath as a stream of white light entering through your nose or mouth and travelling all the way to the bottom of the lungs.

And, on the out breath, imagine dark, acrid smoke.

As you gently breathe in white light, feelings of positivity enter your body and mind. Feel them travel to your extremities.

As you breathe out the dark smoke, you will feel negative thoughts and emotions leave you.

As you continue to do this, you will feel the dark smoke begin to become paler and thinner, suffused by the white light of positivity that is circulating.

Eventually, the smoke becomes difficult to see and every part of your body is filled with light and positivity.

Open your eyes and gently bring yourself back to your current situation with a renewed sense of positivity.

This, and other techniques like it, can be practised at any time, anywhere, and can improve mood and mind-set. Learning to habitually take care of your wellbeing will lead to permanent change.

M5: Cleaning your attic meditation

Specific issues	D F G L M Q
Gap analysis	6 7 8 12 19 20

This meditation helps us to reframe negative thoughts and core beliefs.

Use it when you are processing feedback, recovering from trauma or conflict, and when beginning new projects.

Today is a good day to clean out the attic.

Today you will get to the bottom of the clutter so that you can see the floorboards.

And the walls.

The hidden spaces where the old and unwanted are stored.

Today you will sort out the useful from the obsolete.

You will repair, polish, maybe even modify those things which still serve you.

And you will give away, recycle or throw away anything which you no longer need.

But which is taking up valuable space.

So gather up all of the equipment that you might need.

Dustpans and brushes.

Mops and buckets.

Dusters and cloths.

Large refuse sacks for the removal of unwanted items.

Now, take yourself to a time when you have felt frustrated.

Perhaps very recently.

Or maybe some time ago.

Perhaps a situation which reflects some current sense of unhappiness or discontent.

Maybe a situation at home.

Or in the workplace.

Or it might be something different altogether.

Allow the feelings associated with this to come up to the surface now.

Where do they express themselves in your body?

pause

Now follow these feelings back to their original source.

They do not originate here, in this situation.

But in the thought patterns and core beliefs that you hold deep inside yourself.

Because we each have our own unique model of the world.

Based on our genetic make-up and our unique set of experiences.

This is the lens through which we see the world around us.

Follow the feelings to their *original source*.

And find the negative belief from which they originate.

Ask yourself, 'Is this really true?'

Listen to the answers that come.

Allow yourself to become aware of the part of you that first drew this conclusion.

Know how young you were then.

Allow yourself to come up with an alternative for that belief.

One that *is* true and that serves you much better now.

Let yourself believe it.

Now look around you for all the outmoded beliefs.

And thought and behaviour patterns that no longer serve you.

They suited you at the time that they were created.

But which are now obsolete.

Begin to sweep, dust and clean your attic.

Fill the bin bags with the things that you no longer need.

Make *space*.

Now it is time to gather up the rubbish.

Polish the fixtures and fittings.

And put away your equipment.

Add any finishing touches that you need to.

And leave it as tidy as you would like to find it.
You can tidy up your attic at any time.
It all belongs to you.

M6: Cultivating stillness meditation

Specific issues	A C E R
Gap analysis	2 3 5 7 8 10 15 20

It is in stillness that we can reflect.

Use this meditation to cultivate a mindful state, giving you the time and space to observe and accept events rather than participate in them.

Find a quiet place to sit for a few minutes between tasks.

Take your awareness to the tidal flow of your breath.

Allow it to slow and deepen and notice the feeling of quiet calmness that settles over you.

As you have done before, allow the out breath to become just a little bit longer than the in breath, and notice that familiar feeling of letting go in the body and mind.

Imagine that you have taken precious time out of your day to sit by the ocean.

Look at the sea. Like your breath, there is a hypnotic ebb and flow that occurs naturally, without you having to do anything at all.

Sometimes, the waves crash on to the shore and then pull back with all the force of nature at their back.

Sometimes the water is so calm that it is barely possible to detect the rhythmical shimmer at the water's edge.

Today is a calm day.

Although water ebbs and flows very gently at the edges, the rest of it appears perfectly still.

There is no breeze to disturb the water's surface. There are no ripples at all.

From where you are sitting, you look up at the sky. It appears bright blue. There are only one or two white clouds and, in the sharp light, you can see the moon hovering in the daytime.

As you slowly breathe in the stillness, an awareness comes to you that the moon, the clouds and the bright blue of the sky are perfectly reflected in the water below.

Allow yourself to become perfectly still so that you, like the water, can reflect the beauty of the world around you.

Gently allow yourself to come back to the here and now, bringing with you the stillness that you have created.

M7: Dandelion clock meditation

Specific issues	D F G H L M Q R
Gap analysis	3 4 6 12 15 19 20

This meditation is excellent for releasing attachments to projects or situations, setting intentions and manifestation.

Use this tool for closure after upheavals and when goal setting.

Find a comfortable place to sit where you will not be disturbed.

Sit quietly with your spine straight.

Take your awareness to your breathing.

The tidal in and out of your breath.

Feel the rise and fall of your chest and abdomen as the air enters and then leaves your lungs.

Can you feel your heartbeat?

Now allow those breaths to slow and deepen.

As you breathe in, think of everything that you would like to let go of.

All that has been holding you back.

And as you breathe out, release it.

Blow it back to the universe with gratitude.

You have no use for it now.

Now feel everything around you become quiet and still.

Imagine that you are walking through a wide meadow.

The end of summer is approaching, and weather is warm and balmy.

The sun is at your back and your shadow stretches ahead of you as you make your way through the long grass.

You can hear the birds gossiping in the trees and crickets chirruping around your feet.

All is at peace and in balance.

You unfurl the picnic rug that you have brought with you and place it on the soft ground.

As you sit down to relax, you feel the spring of the grass pushing up beneath the rug to cushion you.

You lie down to drift away for a few moments in the warm sunshine.

When you open your eyes again, you notice a cluster of perfectly whole dandelion clocks.

You marvel at their patterns and symmetry.

As you do so, you begin to see them as pure potential.

Each one boasts row upon row of tiny seeds, waiting to be taken off in a breath of wind.

Every seed is ripe and ready.

Each one is on the cusp of its individual journey.

You wonder if such potential could be harnessed.

As you dreamily watch these complex and intricate marvels of nature, you begin to see what they represent.

Careful not to lose any seeds, you begin by picking the one closest to you.

Each seed on this clock presents as an old, outmoded belief or behaviour that no longer serves you.

On here also are old attachments to mistakes and unpleasant

experiences from which you have learned all there is to
learn.

It is time to let go.

You take a deep breath.

As you blow the dandelion seeds, you whisper:

'I blow you back to the universe. I am grateful for all that
you did for me and all that I learned from you but you no
longer serve me. I release my attachment to you.'

You watch as the seeds float beautifully away on the currents
of air and make their way back to their first source.

You reach to carefully pick another.

Each little seed of potential on this clock represents hopes,
wishes, plans and intentions from all areas of your life.

Some of them are familiar and clearly defined.

Some of them are mere whispers of suggestion, followed by
doubt.

You look very carefully at these seeds.

There are some that you had not noticed until now.

Which ones do you actually want to become *manifest?*

As you examine this clock, you take some time to visualize
where you want each individual seed to go when it breaks
free.

You take a deep breath.

As you blow, you whisper:

'I fully recognize each one of you and know that you all
have the potential to become manifest. I blow each of you
towards your perfect destination according to my wishes
knowing that it is done. I trust the process and release all
my attachment to outcomes.'

Now you watch the seeds fly up in a cloud of stars, visualizing each one as it twirls and eddies along its journey
until it is out of sight.

Just next to the dandelion clocks you see one perfect
dandelion flower.

It is in full bloom.

You pause for a moment, feeling the warmth of the dandelion sun on your face.

After a while, you gently get up from your resting place, pack away your rug and head home.

Making your way back through the meadow in the setting sun, you notice one single buoyant dandelion seed floating along the path ahead.

Now gently bring yourself back to full awareness in the knowledge that you have helped to sow some very important seeds!

M8: Empathy bubble meditation

Specific issues	C D H N P
Gap analysis	4 5 11 12 13 19 20

This meditation helps us to stop absorbing the emotions of others. It also helps to shield us from our triggers while we work on our self-awareness.

Use this meditation regularly to protect yourself from harmful outside influences.

Begin by bringing your attention to your breathing.

Take your awareness to the tidal in and out of your breath.

As you do this, begin to slow and deepen those breaths, taking the air right down into the bottom of your lungs.

And now, as your breath deepens and slows, become aware of the feeling of calm stillness that settles over you.

Now, as you breathe deeply and slowly, just begin to allow the out breath to become just a little bit longer than the in breath.

Deeply and slowly.

It's widely understood that, as we breathe in, the tension in our muscles ever so slightly increases.

And that, as we breathe out, the tension in our bodies relaxes and is let go just a little bit.

So, as you gently deepen and lengthen that out breath, begin to experience that letting go.

Letting go of any tension that you have been holding in your body.

Now set the intention that you are going to protect yourself from any harmful outside influences.

Anything that might have a negative impact on you.

Anything that might drain you or cause you irritation or discomfort.

Now ground yourself.

Imagine roots, like those of a tree, emerging through the souls of your feet and reaching into the soil, connecting you with the earth.

Now imagine a fine silver thread connecting the top of your head with the whole of the cosmos.

And place yourself inside a bubble.

The bubble is warm and light, flexible and buoyant.

It can expand and contract, and it can bend and change shape in the breeze.

Feel its warmth.

Its stillness.

Listen to its silence.

Breathe.

This bubble is made of a very special material which can allow in helpful and useful things.

But it can filter out anything harmful.

Anything which feeds and nourishes your spirit is allowed into the bubble.

But anything that might drain, irritate or upset you simply bounces off and away back to its source.

Inside the bubble, you can be the observer.

The wisest version of yourself.

Here you can observe any situation as it actually is.
Time inside the bubble seems to slow down.
Allowing space between words and thoughts.
And you can see a wider perspective.
A big picture.
And it allows you to act accordingly, in a measured way.
You choose how to respond.
Without being clouded by emotion.
Sit in your bubble and breathe.
Make a deal with yourself to use your bubble.
It's easy to find.
And it is your safe space to use at any time.
Remember to begin with your breathing.
And the rest will follow.

M9: Feather meditation

Specific issues	F G H L M O Q
Gap analysis	3 4 6 12 15 19 20

This meditation is a powerful way to apply the Universal Law of Detachment after setting intentions. It is also a beautiful way to let go of things that are blocking our progress.

Use it for closure, resolution and goal setting.

Find a comfortable place to sit where you will not be disturbed.
This meditation works well when sitting outside in the open.
Sit quietly with your spine straight.
Take your awareness to your breathing.
The tidal in and out of your breath.
Feel the rise and fall of your chest and abdomen as the air enters and then leaves your lungs.
Now allow those breaths to slow and deepen.

And feel everything around you become quiet and still.

Imagine that you are standing at the foot of a beautiful mountain.

The end of summer is approaching, and the weather is warm and balmy.

The sun is high in the blue sky and a gentle breeze whispers as you make your way through the long, tufty grass to begin your ascent.

You can hear birds of prey keening as they climb the thermal currents way above your head, and the playful sound of bubbling water from the brook running down the mountain side.

All is at peace and in balance.

As you look down at your feet, you notice a beautiful, coloured feather.

You reach down and collect it.

It reflects every colour.

Iridescent in the sunlight.

You begin to steadily climb.

The atmosphere is warm and alive, and the exercise is exhilarating.

As you reach the halfway point, you notice that the air is becoming fresher and cooler.

The change is welcome.

The gentle breeze has become a steady wind.

Blowing away anything that has stayed with you for too long.

You stop and allow the wind to blow you in all directions.

As you do this, you take your awareness to anything that you wish to be free of.

Any old belief, outmoded thought pattern or unwanted behaviour that has outstayed its welcome.

Maybe some things that were useful once but no longer serve you now.

Even as you bring them into your awareness.

They are immediately taken up by the air and blown away, back to source.

Renewing your sense of Self.

Freeing you and leaving you lighter.

And ready to complete your ascent.

As you continue to climb, you notice the wind growing stronger and stronger.

You marvel at its enormous energy.

It buffets you in all directions.

You can also see the place you left behind becoming smaller and smaller.

Enabling you to see *all* of it.

The bigger picture.

Everything in its place and everything in balance.

The bird's-eye view.

Now, as you reach the top of this giant mountain, you feel the wind roaring around your ears.

You are almost lifted up by its strength.

The view below is astonishing.

You can see *everything*.

What seemed difficult before seems logical and easy now.

Like pieces of a jigsaw puzzle.

As you stand and feel the full force of the wind.

You take out your feather.

You hold it between your fingertips and fill it with *all* your ideas.

Your hopes.

Your intentions.

Your ambitions.

Every seed of creativity that has expressed itself within you now comes into your awareness.

Things that you have wanted to try but have been held back from by fear.

Breathe *all* of them into your feather.
Ready to be given life.
When you are ready, let it go.
Watch as the strong currents of air pick it up.
Twirl it and dance with it.
Higher and higher.
Until it disappears.
Entrusted to the universe for right action.
Now detach yourself from old feelings of disappointment.
Let go of need and resentment.
Know that they only block your progress.
Allow yourself to soak up the energy of this great wind.
To feel the steadiness of the earth beneath your feet as you
    soar like the birds of prey.
When you are ready.
Begin to make your gentle descent.
Lighter and energized.
Back to full awareness with a brand-new perspective.

M10: Flow meditation

Specific issues	D F G H R S
Gap analysis	3 5 14 16 17

*This tool is about being open to receive all things, and being able to
let them go to avoid stagnation. Holding on to things means we may
have no room for new opportunities.*

Use this tool regularly to maintain flow.

Whatever comes to you flows through you and on.

El Morya

As always, take your awareness to your breathing.
Appreciate its tidal quality.

And the constant renewal of clean, refreshed air that you are
supplied with.

Slow, steady and adaptable.

This is *flow*.

Allow the breath to slow and deepen, just as you have done
many times before.

Recognize the feeling of calm that settles over you.

Imagine that you are out for a walk.

On a beautiful summer day.

There is a slight breeze.

And summer is in full bloom.

The air is warm.

And the gentle wind carries to you all the scents of nature.

In the distance you can hear water.

From far off there is a rushing sound.

But much closer you hear the gentle babbling and splashing
of a large stream.

As you walk towards the sound, it comes into view.

A sunlit stream where the water flows.

At such a pace that it is neither a gushing torrent nor a
snaking green slick.

Neither too fast.

Or too slow.

As you approach, the water seems to jump and dance in the
sunlight.

Reflecting every colour of the rainbow.

You crouch down at the edge of the stream.

And reach your hand into the water.

It is surprisingly warm and incredibly inviting.

So you take off your shoes and socks.

And step into the stream.

The feeling of the water is so pleasant.

And the water is deep enough for you to sit down.

Before you know it, you are lying down in the clear, iridescent water.

Allowing it to flow through your hair and clothes.

Refreshing every fibre of your being.

As you lie there in the water.

You watch the white fluffy clouds drift overhead.

Although you are completely still in the water, you feel that you, too, are drifting.

With the gentle bob and flow of the water around you.

Somewhere upstream is a stagnant pond.

And downstream is a gushing torrent.

But here the flow is steady and constant.

New and pleasant water coming.

And then leaving.

Constantly renewing.

Unchanging, but *ever* changing.

As you lie in the water, you begin to visualize your joys.

Your pain.

Your successes.

Your regrets.

Your happiness.

Your sadness.

Everything that has come and gone.

And you appreciate the flow of the water all around you.

Bringing the joys and the lessons.

But always moving forward.

Alleviating discomfort.

Dissolving doubt.

Melting away pain.

Bringing creativity.

New growth.

And the constant renewal of all things.

You allow yourself to be bathed in hope and gratitude.

You lie there for a while.

Bathing in the flow of the water.

As you leave the stream, you are refreshed and renewed.

Ready to face whatever comes your way.

Gently bring yourself back to full awareness with a renewed sense of hope and positivity. Remember, always, to immerse yourself in life's flow.

M11: Gratitude meditation

SUPERTOOL

Specific issues	A–T
Gap analysis	1–20

It is all too easy, when visualizing where we want to be, to focus our thoughts on what we need rather than what we already have. This occurs when we perceive that we should be moving towards our goals and we are concentrating on the prize. By doing this, we are driven by lack and become indifferent to everything that has already been gifted to us.

Acknowledging the gifts offered to us in all situations, whether positive or negative, allows us to create a grateful mind-set. This activates the Universal Law of Attraction, which, in turn, creates abundance.

Practise this universal gratitude meditation as part of your regular Self-care regime.

Find a quiet place where you will not be disturbed.

Sit in a comfortable position with your spine straight.

Take your awareness to your breathing.

The tidal in and out of your breath.

Allow it to slow and deepen.

Become aware of the stillness that settles over you.

Be grateful for that stillness.

Become aware of the vibrant life force that is your body.

Feel your heartbeat.

Every cell nourished.

Every sensation registered.

The joy of sight.

Sound. Smell. Taste. Touch.

And movement.

Your body *speaks* to you.

And it *listens*.

Allow yourself to become grateful for the freedom that this affords you.

And the opportunities it brings.

See yourself at rest in your usual surroundings.

Picture your home.

All the things that you have surrounded yourself with.

For comfort and convenience.

Collected over time.

Things with meaning.

Style. Elegance and function.

Picture all the physical possessions that you value.

However small.

With their different and varied uses and purposes.

Recognize and acknowledge each one in turn.

And allow the process to invoke *gratitude*.

Let it flow.

Now picture yourself in your positive relationships.

With loved ones.

Family members.

Friends. Colleagues. Animals.

Picture each relationship one by one.

All of them complex. Multifaceted.

And unique.

Feel the love.

Friendship.

Camaraderie.

Support.

And compassion.

These things easily invoke gratitude.

Allow it to *rise up*.

Now see yourself in the relationships which present you with challenges.

Learning tough lessons.

Addressing misunderstanding.

Practising negotiation and compromise.

Being uncomfortably provoked so that you can see where you need to work on your Self.

These are gifts of *resilience*.

Thank those relationships.

Give that gratitude time for it to come to the surface.

Know that, without them, the lessons would be lost.

Now picture all your life events and lessons.

Big or small.

Positive or negative.

Everything you learned.

From being taught.

Or through your experiences.

Every situation, however difficult, has something valuable to teach you.

About the Self.

Without those experiences, the lessons would be lost.

Allow yourself to be grateful for those, too.

They make up your model of the world.

Decide now to view every day with the same level of gratitude.

To allow every experience.

No matter how small it seems.

That may otherwise have passed unnoticed.

To be *acknowledged* for the gifts it can offer you.

How does that feel?

Now gently bring yourself back to full awareness.

Refreshed and bathed in gratitude.

M12: Ocean meditation

Specific issues	A B C E R S
Gap analysis	2 14 15 16 17 20

This meditation is fantastic for anxiety and stepping back from any situation that is causing distress.

Use it when recovering from trauma or conflict, when you feel anxious or unsupported and adrift.

Take your awareness to your breathing.

The tidal in and out of your breath.

As you do this, begin to allow that breath to slow and deepen.

Deeply and slowly.

Become aware of the feeling of calm that settles over you.

And now begin to allow the out breath to become just a little bit longer than the in breath.

It's widely accepted that, as we breathe in, we experience a little rise in tension in our bodies.

And that, as we breathe out, we are able to let that tension go.

Now picture yourself taking a walk by the sea.

It is sunrise and you are the only person who has taken the time to get up to take in this precious moment.

And it is yours.

The air is warm and balmy and you are calm and centred.

A few of the night stars are still pricking the dawn sky.

Which contains all the colours of the new day approaching.

As you step on to the sand, turn and begin to make your way along the beach.

Along the shoreline.

Your awareness is drawn to the rhythmical rush of the waves.

Rolling forward.

And drawing back.

So you pause and look out towards the horizon.

And you take a moment to breathe in the sea air.

You take in the salt scent of the sea.

And become connected.

As your breath begins to slow and deepen once more.

You realize that it matches the rhythmical motion of the waves.

You are one with the sea.

And the earth, and early-morning sky.

Now pause to look at the ocean.

Become an observer.

The ocean has many moods.

Sometimes the waves are crashing wildly in.

A raging torrent of power and motion.

Sometimes they are a trickle of skipping water.

Emerging from a calm, flat sea.

But it is always the ocean.

When you stand and observe the ocean.

You can appreciate its diversity.

Its breath-taking beauty.

And the immensely powerful forces contained within it.

Without becoming consumed by them.

You can stand back.

Now watch as the sun begins to rise over the sea.

Filling the sky with colour and light.

With it, the whole body of water becomes calm and still.

Except for the gentle ebbing and flowing at the shoreline.

Rolling forward.

And drawing back.

At one with your breath.

And, with that, you turn from the sea and head home.

Taking with you a perfect sense of peace.

M13: Rise meditation

Specific issues	A B C D F G Q S
Gap analysis	3 4 5 19 20

This meditation helps to detach from everything that weighs us down. It also allows us to see ourselves without our unwanted baggage.

Use this meditation for letting go of fears, negative thoughts and core beliefs, attachments to situations, labels and pain, unburdening the Self to free up energy for creativity.

When we are attached to human sensibilities we cannot RISE!

Sit quietly in your chair, close your eyes.

And breathe in and out, deeply and effortlessly.

Follow the air right to the bottom of your lungs and notice how the letting go of it encourages a letting go in the rest of your body.

Notice the little noises around you.

The ebb and flow of life as the world carries on.

Without you for these few moments.

Picture yourself walking through dense woodland on a warm, spring morning.

As the sun gently pierces the protective canopy of trees.

It warms the still, forest air and releases the heady, fresh scent of the trees.

Tiny creatures scurry for cover at the sound of you approaching.

And high in the branches, birds and insects chirrup in celebration of a new day.

The journey is so pleasant that you pay no attention to its length or purpose.

It is enough just to *be* in the woods.

Among the plants and creatures that live there.

After you have been walking for a while.

A large clearing seems to appear out of nowhere.

And you step out into bright, warm sunlight.

To the sound of whispering trees.

And another sound which you cannot quite make out.

A soft and gentle rustling from farther away.

At the other side of the clearing, you can see a large fluid object.

Shimmering in the sunlight.

And gently billowing in the breeze.

As you walk towards it, you realize that it is a hot-air balloon.

Shifting restlessly just above the clearing floor.

As you move closer, you can see its magnificent silks, shuddering and trembling with anticipation.

The balloon's basket is open, and you are able to climb inside.

By lifting the silks and crawling underneath them.

The light, exquisite fabric is delicate and soft on your skin.

And you make yourself comfortable among the soft, pretty cushions and rugs.

As you do this, suddenly a huge white flame appears in its centre.

Away from where you are sitting.

It has been waiting for you to enter.

The balloon is instantly filled with heat and upward movement.

It is filled with your creative fire.

It is also tugging at the ropes that hold it fast.

It wants to go.

To RISE.

Now you are able to look around and peer outside, over the edge of the little basket.

You curiously notice that the ropes that hold the balloon fast to the ground are attached to bags, bottles and cases of various different sizes and shapes.

Some are small and easily rocked by the motion of the balloon; others are large and heavy.

As you examine these bags, you notice that each one has a label.

One reads *guilt*. One, *resentment*. Another, *regret*. As you continue to read the labels, you see many that you recognize. *Poor body-image, low self-worth* and so on.

On reading the labels you begin to see that these are the things that you must let go of in order to RISE. *Old arguments. Outmoded beliefs* and *ideas* which no longer serve you. *Old expectations* of yourself and others. *Visions of how things should have been* that have not come to pass.

Take out whatever tools you have brought with you and begin to work at the ropes. Some of them will loosen more easily than others.

When the first rope is unwound and separated from the basket, you feel a visceral lurching upwards as the balloon frees itself from that one piece of baggage.

It catches again, though, as the other ropes that still hold it become taut once more. But each time you loosen one of the ropes, the balloon pushes upwards towards the sky.

You work methodically around the edge of the basket, untying, disentangling and even cutting the ropes that remain, each time feeling the lurch towards freedom – until, finally, the last knot is undone!

You barely notice the upwards motion, just the earth beneath you becoming smaller and smaller and the ropes and bags falling away.

And now you are free.

You RISE!

Up and away.

With pure intention as your compass, you RISE towards your purpose in the currents of air, powered by your own creative fire.

Gently drift back towards the earth when you are ready. Watch as, effortlessly, the balloon finds the little clearing in the woods and slowly, purposefully, descends to land softly, exactly where you found it, ready for your next adventure.

When you are ready, open your eyes and return to your earthly situation. Now you can enjoy the rest of your day with renewed peace and a lighter outlook.

When you detach from what has been holding you down, YOU RISE!

M14: Roost on the wing meditation

Specific issues	A B C H S
Gap analysis	1 2 5 8 13 20

This meditation is for creating peace at any time, particularly during a busy day.

Use it as part of your regular Self-care regimen and when you feel overwhelmed, stressed or in pain.

Find a space where you can sit or lie comfortably.

Begin by becoming aware of your breathing.

Become your breath as it rises and falls.

Slowly.

In and out.

Now allow the out breath to become longer than the in breath.

Watch it lengthen.

It's easy when you let go.

And, with every in breath, breathe in positive thoughts and good feelings.

And, with every out breath, let go of any negativity.

Focus only on your breath.

You have all the time in the world.

As you focus on your breathing, allow yourself to become light.

Your thoughts are light.

Your body is light.

You are weightless and you can float safely, high above the ground.

Anything that is weighing you down can be left here at the edge of your mat to be collected later.

Or not.

Take yourself back to a time when you felt under pressure.

Maybe from the demands of work.

Deadlines.

Expectations of others.

Perhaps family.

Trying to find a balance.

Or any other external source.

A time when you have felt stretched to capacity.

Overloaded.

Unable to bear the weight.

Allow those feelings to fully come to the surface.

Where do they express themselves in your body?

Can you name them?

Now let them dissolve away.

You know, there are birds that can roost on the wing.

They can stay up in the air for up to ten months at a time.

Swooping and soaring high above the earth.

Catching flies.

Feeding their young.

Travelling in numbers.

Organized and ordered.

But spontaneous and adaptive.

They have all the skills and tools they need for a long-haul flight.

Right there.

It is in them.

They cannot afford to come down and rest between destinations.

They do not wish to.

They need their focus for the long journey.

But they need to arrive rested and refreshed.

So they keep a steady pace.

And, rather than coming down to rest, they take rest up with them.

Into the air.

They roost on the wing.

Because they are experts in their craft.

Like you, they have spent long days learning.

Acquiring those very specific skills.

Honing them.

Practising with their brothers and sisters.

Becoming masters of their art.

So that it becomes almost automatic.

Unconscious.

It is instinct.

They don't think about those skills.

It is who they are.

Wheeling and soaring above the clouds.

Climbing the thermals and diving through the air.

Protecting and nurturing their young and old.

Nourishing and sustaining themselves and each other.

Roosting and resting.

Bringing peace to their journey.

As you breathe in deeply and easily.

Letting go of any negativity on your out breath.

Breathe in that travelling peace.

A peace which can exist anywhere.

Peace which does not require the stopping of everything else.

Or the interruption of the dance of life.

Breathe in the peace of roosting on the wing.
And take it with you.

pause

Now let those images dissolve and fade.
But know that those pleasant, restful feelings can remain.
As you come slowly and gently back to full awareness.
And know that you can take peace with you.
Steadying the pace.
You can work and rest at the same time.
And arrive rested and refreshed.
As you roost on the wing.

M15: Shower meditation

Specific issues	D G L M Q R
Gap analysis	3 4 6 7 12 13 19 20

Water is a means of travel in the physical world. It is also widely used symbolically in meditative visualization and shamanic journeying.

We use water on a daily basis to cleanse ourselves and our environment. Our daily cleansing rituals undoubtedly have advantages that go far beyond the physical. We all know the benefits of an energizing shower before work, or a relaxing soak in the bath at the end of a long day. What if we made this process more conscious?

What if we set our intention to further enhance our daily water rituals?

Use this tool to habitually cleanse yourself of what does not serve you, and bathe in what nourishes you.

Think about your daily encounters with water.
Showering in the morning before work.
Washing your hands throughout the day.
Maybe going for a swim.
Taking a long soak in the bath in the evening to relax.

As you prepare to do these activities, set the intention to do them *mindfully.*

It is possible to let your physical body take care of things automatically, while you are taking a shower or washing your hands. This means that you are free to become a prisoner to your thoughts, and not be present during the process at all.

When we set our intention to become present, we can harness the power of water and its symbolic value.

As you step into the shower or bath, or place your hands under running water today, silently say to yourself:

'I cleanse myself of anything I am attached to that no longer serves me.'

'I cleanse myself of negative thoughts and feelings.'

'I cleanse myself of self-criticism and judgement.'

'I bathe myself in new growth and progress.'

'I bathe myself in positive thoughts and feelings.'

I bathe myself in acceptance and gratitude.'

You can visualize as the things that you have been holding on to, that no longer serve you, flow away down the plug hole. As you do this, allow the fresh, clean water to bathe you in positivity and light.

As you begin to make this your ritual, you may well find that more appropriate words and phrases arrive. Let the mantra become your own. Your higher Self knows the words that will resonate with you and benefit you the most.

Whenever I am near water, I cleanse myself of what no longer fits for me, and bathe in what serves me. I do this with gratitude and acceptance.

M16: Spiral meditation

Specific issues	D F G H L M Q R
Gap analysis	3 4 6 12 15 19 20

This meditation is for endings and beginnings. It is for letting go of things that no longer serve us and creating a new perspective.

Use this at the end or beginning of a project – think about what you want to let go of and what you want to take forward.

Find a quiet, comfortable place where you will not be disturbed.

Sit, relaxed, with your spine straight.

Take your awareness to your breathing as you have done before.

The tidal in and out of your breath.

Aligning with all the cycles, patterns and symmetry of the natural world.

The rolling sea.

The Earth as it orbits the Sun.

The flower as it bursts silently open.

Quickened by the warmth of summer sunshine.

Allow your shoulders to soften.

Allow your breath to become slow and deep.

Picture yourself walking along a cliff top on a warm spring morning.

You can hear the sound of the seabirds calling from far offshore.

And you notice the scent of sea salt in the new morning air.

As you begin your descent towards the shoreline.

Making your way along the sloping path downwards.

You notice tufts of coarse sea grass, stirring in the breeze.

And tiny buzzing insects, holding fast in the undergrowth.

Your feet keep a steady rhythm until, at last, they find the flat expanse of damp sand.

That stretches out towards the foaming water's edge.

You walk along the beach.

Listening to the lap, lap, lap of the tiny waves eddying over the sand.

Way off in the distance you can see a disturbance of colour
and texture.

Along the flat expanse of beach.

You make your way curiously towards it.

Taking in its variety of subtle dotting of pink, blue, green
and gold.

It is a large stone sea birds.

Perfectly made.

Beautifully designed.

The colours and textures are random.

And yet, somehow, uniform.

It is walkable!

With gratitude, you put down your bag.

Take off your shoes and socks.

And allow the warm wet sand between your toes.

You close your eyes.

And breathe deeply the salty morning air.

You ask yourself:

'What do I carry today that no longer serves me?'

'What do I wish to let go of?'

The answers seem to arrive on the wind.

Holding those answers gently between your fingers and thumb.

You begin to walk the spiral inwards, towards the centre.

Conscious of each turn representing all the changes.

You have both accepted and resisted.

In the passing of the years.

When you reach the centre of the spiral.

You picture those things that no longer serve you.

Held gently between your fingers and thumb.

And you release them into the wind.

You say:

'I release the things that were once mine.

But that no longer serve me or nourish my spirit.

I let them go in the breeze.

To be blown gently back to source.'

You stand there in the centre of the beautiful spiral.

And let go.

Opening your fingers and thumbs.

And allowing all that you brought to be released.

To flutter and drift away on the wind.

Like feathers.

And now you ask yourself:

'What do I wish to take with me for the journey ahead?'

'What will nourish me and bolster me in my new and current ventures?'

'What do I wish to cultivate and nurture to give me support and sustenance?'

The answers arrive on the wind.

You press them gently to your heart.

Taking them as your own.

Knowing that they are a gift.

After some time, you begin slowly walking the spiral outwards.

Towards the undisturbed sand.

Holding your gifts closely and safely within.

Each turn representing limitless potential and growth.

In your rhythmical walking, you begin to see how these gifts will be used.

To support and assist you.

In your journey forwards.

From this point onwards.

And you are filled with gratitude.

And hope.

And joy.

Now your journey begins anew.

The next full turn.

As you make the steady climb to the top of the cliff.

Now gently bring yourself back to full awareness.

Feeling refreshed and ready to face the rest of the day.

M17: The White Room mindfulness meditation

SUPERTOOL

Specific issues	A–T
Gap analysis	1–20

This meditation helps us to experience mindfulness. Coming into true presence can allow us to address any difficulty within our life, making this a universal tool. By accepting that the only power we have is in the present moment, we can take any appropriate action in the now and accept what cannot be changed.

Use your white room regularly to practise mindfulness.

Find a comfortable place to sit with your spine straight.

Take your awareness to your breathing.

The tidal in and out of your breath.

Allow it to slow and deepen.

Feel a sense of calm settle over you.

Place yourself in the centre of a white room.

The room is empty, spacious and comfortable.

You are calm and centred.

In the white room is only the present moment.

The here and the now.

Nothing else resides here.

It's very important for you to remember that this place.

Of the present.

Of the here and now.

This white room.

Is the only place where you have actual power.

Because it is the present moment.

Here is where the future is determined by current thought.

As you sit in the centre of the white room, you will notice a door to the right of you.

Behind this door lies the future.

But it is a future of infinite possibilities and limitless potential.

It is unknowable.

Free of any constraints.

Free of past conditioning.

And limiting beliefs.

Worrying about future events, be it tomorrow or years from now, is not appropriate.

You cannot step through the door because the future is not determined yet.

You determine the future with the thoughts, beliefs and intentions that you hold right here in the present.

In the white room you are the *architect* of the future.

What thoughts belong here?

What seeds do you want to plant?

And in the white room there is a door to the left of you.

Behind it is the past.

Everything that has ever happened, right from childhood.

Up until just a few moments ago.

Every memory.

Every thought, feeling, emotion.

Every action or inaction that has shaped your model of the world up to now.

All on the other side of the door.

You cannot step through this door either.

Because it is known.

It is limited by past conditioning and beliefs.

It is unchangeable.

Sometimes thoughts drift through these doors into the white room.

Thoughts about the future.

Perhaps worrying about a meeting at work.

Whether a task will be completed on time.

Thoughts about the past.

Perhaps recalling a conversation with someone.

Or reliving an experience.

Good or bad.

Pleasant or unpleasant.

Sometimes they drift through the door.

But nothing resides here.

Except the present.

You.

In this room.

Listening.

Now take a few moments to examine the thoughts that are circling *your* white room.

If it is a future concern.

Like your plans for tomorrow.

A future appointment, or an even unknown.

Give it a label.

And put it through the door to the right.

If it's a past concern.

Like a conversation from last week or your journey home from work.

Something that's already happened.

Give it a label.

And put it behind the door to the left.

As you sit in the white room today.

Feel that there is infinite potential here.

Be grateful for the power to choose what you bring into this space.

And to keep it free of anything that does not belong.

Remember, you can check the contents of your white room at any time.

At work.

In the evening.

During the night.

Keep it tidy and use it well.

It all belongs to you.

M18: The White Room for crisis meditation

Specific issues	A B E F H N R (in acute examples of these specific issues)
Gap analysis	15 20

This tool is adapted from M17: The White Room mindfulness meditation. It helps us to create some space for the processing of information and helps us to manage the intense emotions felt when something terrible has happened or when we are in crisis.

Use this tool when you feel overwhelmed by your current situation.

Place yourself in the centre of your white room.

It is spacious and comfortable.

You are calm and centred.

It is a place of the here and now.

The present moment.

Nothing else can reside here.

Breathe deeply and allow all the emotions brought about by the current situation to come to the surface.

Every feeling.

Every sensation.

Physical and emotional.

Let them all be present here in all of their complexity.

What does it feel like?

Where do they express themselves in your body?

Now allow all of the thoughts that are dominating this space to be heard.

Thoughts that have come through the doors to the right and left of you.

Reliving the receipt of news or imparting it.

Pain.

Grief.

Fears about others.

Imaginings of events to come.
Give them all space in here.
Allow them to flow.
Do not resist them.

pause

Now step into the shoes of your Observer Self.
And bear witness to what is here.
However complex.
Unexpected.
Uninvited.
Unwanted.
Unpleasant.
Whatever else this is, it is a learning situation.
An opportunity to sharpen your skills through adversity.
Your chance to prepare for the future.
The unknowable.
Bring your awareness to your breathing.
Now slowly begin to label each component of the situation.
One by one.
Every thought.
Positive or negative.
Good or bad.
Every feeling and emotion.
Physical or otherwise.
One by one.
Label them and examine which door they should be stored
    behind.
Only for the moment.
In a place where they can be easily retrieved.
Because they are necessary for your healing.
And you will need to be able to access them.
One by one.
In your own time.

Gently label them and sort them.

Just behind the door to the right.

Or the door to the left.

Now breathe into this space you have created.

Fill your lungs.

Relax your body.

Now place a glass screen up in front of you.

It is an impenetrable screen of tough, clear glass.

You can see through it clearly.

At the other side of the screen is the white room with its doors.

To the right and the left.

Behind which you have stored all of the components of this situation.

Now you are able to allow the thoughts and emotions that you have labelled.

Back through the doors into the white room.

But behind this screen you can only observe.

The emotions do not affect you in the same way.

You are aware of them but they have lost their intensity.

They appear more ordered.

You can sort them further.

And now there is space in between them.

There is also *understanding*.

And *acceptance*.

Now sort all of those components of the situation again.

Storing them just through the doors to the right and left of you.

It is easier this time.

pause

Breathe deeply again.

In this space.

In the white room is the present moment.

The here and now.

This is your breathing space.

Now you can remove your glass screen because you no longer
   need it.

For now, in the present.

In your white room.

There is space.

And only what is happening right now.

You.

In this room.

But when you choose to allow those thoughts and emotions.

That you have stored and labelled behind the doors.

Back into the white room for processing.

Their intensity will be manageable.

There will be order.

There will be acceptance.

And the space for you to be calm and centred.

And you will be able to process them accordingly.

Leaving your white room tidy and clear.

For you to manifest the most positive outcome that the
   situation will allow.

Through current thought.

It is your space.

It belongs to you.

M19: Tree meditation

Specific issues	A B J K S
Gap analysis	5 6 7 16 17

This is a great meditation for cultivating health and vitality by connecting with the body. This is a beautiful meditation to do as a treat!

   Use this as part of your Self-care regimen, if you are not feeling well or if you need a boost.

Take your awareness to your breathing once again.

The tidal in and out of your breath.

Allow it to slow and deepen.

Now be aware of your life force.

Your body hums with vitality.

Your breath.

The beating of your heart.

The blood taking its course through your veins.

Supplying every cell with the energy that it needs.

For you to be alive.

Feel that energy.

Picture it in your body.

See it, bright and vibrant.

Now see it extending beyond your body.

Out into what you call your personal space.

That safe, intimate space around you.

Your place in the universe.

Now picture, in front of you, a beautiful tree.

Out in the beautiful natural world.

See it clearly rooted in the earth.

Reaching to the sky.

Feel its silent knowing.

Its immense sense of presence.

Now unpack a blanket and cushion and sit in its shade.

From here you can close your eyes and lean back against the
      sturdy trunk and let it take your weight.

Take your awareness now to the roots of this tree.

Their connection to the earth.

Follow them deep down into the soil.

This is where the tree draws up all its nutrients.

How do these roots appear to you?

Are they strong?

Do they reach deeply into the ground?

How is it that they can draw up exactly what is needed?

Do what you need to do to strengthen these roots.

Now take your awareness to the trunk and branches of this beautiful tree.

What communication systems lie within?

Are there clear channels for transport there?

Or do you see some blockages?

Put your energy into removing these blockages, however it needs to be done.

When the elements are strong, do the branches bend or break?

Give the tree what it needs to allow it to adapt to the wind.

Give it flexibility.

Now look at the leaves of the tree.

This is the very breath of life itself.

Are they green and lush and wide?

Do they need cleaner air?

Cleanse them now with a mountain breeze.

Do they need water?

Give it to them.

Is there blossom on your tree?

What colour is it?

Breathe in its beauty.

Are there animals or insects?

What is their purpose?

Look at your tree as a whole being of life now.

What can you do to help it to flourish?

Do you need to remove some old wood or spotted leaves?

Can you give it water or nutrients?

Do this now in whatever way feels right to you.

Watch it grow.

Watch as the leaves on your tree reach up to the heavens, connecting it with the cosmos.

Now imagine a silver thread from the top of your head connecting you, forever, to the source of all of our being.

And now begin to slowly allow those images to fade.

Gently.

Yawn. Stretch.

Open your eyes.

M20: Walking meditation

Specific issues	B H S T
Gap analysis	5 7 16 17

Mindful walking is an excellent way to develop a sense of connection with nature and the living world. It is also an excellent way to experience the present moment. Listen to this guided meditation when you take time outside.

Use this tool when you are feeling disconnected.

Step outside and head to a place of quiet solitude.

Walk towards a place where nature is evident.

It could be a forest, river or mountain.

Or it could simply be a tree or some potted plants in your backyard.

Slow your walking pace and take your awareness to your breathing.

The tidal in and out of your breath.

Be conscious of the life-giving in breath that you share with all living things.

And allow the release of the out breath to help you to be free of anything that no longer serves you.

Know that your body has its own cycles and rhythms.

Your body is made of earth material.

Day turns to night and night to day.

The moon waxes and becomes full.

And then wanes to darkness.

The earth, too, has breath.

Take your awareness to your feet.

Feel the firm earth pushing up to meet them.

Feel the connection with the earth.

And all living things.

Pause and imagine your connection with the earth as little roots sprouting from the bottoms of your feet and burrowing down into the fertile soil.

Become in tune with your senses.

Become completely aware of your surroundings in the present moment.

Notice what is beautiful.

And practise gratitude.

Take your awareness to the top of your head.

And the sky beyond.

Far up above you there are planets and stars.

You are a part of it all.

Imagine your celestial connection as vibrant rays of warm light reaching up from the top of your head towards the cosmos.

And in the centre.

One single silver thread.

If thoughts of past or future invade.

Just gently bring yourself back to this moment in time.

It is yours to enjoy right now.

Honour your relationship with everything in the natural world.

Recognize its beauty.

A sense of oneness.

If you have time, sit for a few minutes and be still.

Know your surroundings but rise above your thoughts and just *be*.

And when you are ready, bring yourself back to full awareness with a renewed sense of connection.

M21: Waterfall meditation

Specific issues	A B F J K S
Gap analysis	5 6 7 16 17 20

This meditation, adapted from 'The Waterfall' by Dorothy Lewis,[1] is a powerful way to cleanse and energize.

Use this either at the beginning or end of the day, when recovering from trauma or conflict, and during (or when recovering from) illness.

Take your awareness to your breathing once again.

The tidal in and out of your breath.

Allow it to slow and deepen as you have done before.

Now be aware of your life force.

Your body hums with vitality.

Your breath.

The beating of your heart.

The blood taking its course through your veins.

Supplying every cell with the energy that it needs.

For you to be alive.

Feel that energy.

Picture it in your body.

See it, bright and vibrant.

Now see it extending beyond your body.

Out into what you call your personal space.

That safe, intimate space around you.

Your place in the universe.

Now picture, in front of you, a beautiful waterfall.

Out in the beautiful natural world.

See it clearly, glistening in the sun.

Hear the tremendous rushing of water back to source.

Feel its immense energy.

Its sense of purpose.

Now notice how the misting of the water, as it connects with the earth, has created a huge, beautiful rainbow.

Vibrant in its colour.

Everything about it is energy and light.

Now step into the water and allow it to flow over you.

Cleansing and healing.

Taking away old patterns of behaviour.

And negative thinking.

Flushing them away.

Transmuting and taking them back to source.

Renewing your positivity and vitality.

Recharging you with hope and purpose.

Now step out of the water and into the rainbow.

Let the colour energy blend with your energy.

Let it fill your personal space.

Flow through you.

First, see the red of poppies and your own vital blood.

Now the orange of tangerines and pumpkins.

Warming and energizing you.

Now the beautiful, peaceful yellow of a daffodil.

And the sun itself, with all its power.

Now see all the greens of nature coming to nourish and help you to feel alive.

And the turquoise of the all-vast blue oceans to help you to express yourself clearly.

Now see the deep blues of the summer skies and dragonflies for clarity and precision.

And violet, amethyst and all the purples of the sky after sunset.

Now imagine a silver thread from the top of your head connecting you forever to the source of all of our being.

Breathe in this beauty.

And gently and slowly allow these images to fade, and begin to recall your surroundings with a renewed state of being.

20

Visualization exercises

V1: Anchor positive emotions

Specific issues	A B C F H R S T
Gap analysis	2 15 16 17 19 20

This NLP exercise can be used to anchor a positive emotion to a physical point on the body. This means that it can be quickly retrieved and re-experienced to replace unpleasant emotions by 'firing the anchor' in times of distress.

Before you begin, focus on the type of emotion that you want to evoke. Try to recall a memory where the desired emotion was most evident. It may be your happiest memory, the one where you felt most loved, or the proud memory of your highest achievement.

Next, choose an accessible place on your body where you can easily and subtly press to anchor the emotion. For example, just above your knee or a point on your other hand.

Sit with a straight spine in a quiet space where you will not
   be disturbed.
Be present.
To do this, take your awareness to your breathing.
Allow it to slow and deepen.
Allow your body and mind to become relaxed as you focus
   on the rhythmical in and out of your breath.
Take a few minutes to enjoy the silence.
Now set your intention.

You are going to recall your chosen memory in as much
detail as possible.

Begin to recall it as if it is happening right now.

Visualize it as clearly as you can.

Recalling every single detail, however small.

Remember to call in your other senses.

Recall the sounds.

What is being said to you? Is there music?

Recall smell and taste.

Now recall how it *felt*.

Begin with your body sensations.

Are there butterflies in your stomach?

Is your heart racing?

Now *feel* all the emotion that comes flooding into your
awareness.

Turn it up as brightly and vividly as you can.

Let yourself be *full*.

Now firmly press the spot you have chosen for your anchor.

Hold for a few seconds while you keep recalling the feeling.

Now release, open your eyes, blink, and immediately think of
something unrelated.

Perhaps your next meal.

After a few moments, test the anchor by pressing it again.

Feel those emotions return.

If you want to increase the intensity, you can repeat the process.

V2: Balancing visualization

SUPERTOOL

Specific issues	A–T
Gap analysis	1–20

*This tool grounds, connects and uplifts. It is a universal visualization
technique. Use it habitually throughout the day, before important
events and if you are feeling unsettled.*

Sit comfortably with your spine straight and feet flat on the floor.

Take your awareness to your breathing.

Now imagine roots emerging from the soles of your feet.

Reaching down deeply into the earth.

Feel the connection.

Notice the flow of energy.

Feel rooted and grounded to the earth.

And connected to every living thing.

Know that the deeper you are rooted, the better able you are to withstand the wind.

Now take your awareness to the crown of your head.

Imagine a fine, glistening silver thread.

Right in the centre.

Reaching up into the heavens.

Connecting you with the entire cosmos.

Feel the connection.

Notice the flow of energy.

The Sun, planets, moons and stars.

And everything beyond.

Your unbreakable connection to the universe.

And its boundless potential.

Now feel the abundance of energy that is yours.

If you can be open to receive it.

Set your intention to receive all that is yours.

Gently bring yourself back to full awareness.

V3: Blackboard technique for insomnia

Specific issues	A I R
Gap analysis	3 7

This is a visualization exercise for insomnia. It is adapted from a hypnotherapy script.[1] Use it at night when attempting to fall asleep and also in returning to sleep after you wake in the night.

Begin by imagining a blackboard.

Be specific.

Is your blackboard square or rectangular?

What colour is it?

Let it fill your mind.

On the ledge at the bottom, within easy reach, are a board rubber and a piece of chalk.

Now take the chalk in your hand and choose a corner of the blackboard.

I wonder which corner you will choose.

Now write in that corner, the word *sleep*.

Now take the board rubber and rub out the word that you have written.

Now take the chalk and write, in the middle of the board, the number 1.

Write it as a number rather than a word.

Now take the board rubber and rub out the number 1.

Now choose a corner of the black board and write the word *sleep*.

Perhaps you will choose the same corner; perhaps you will pick another.

Maybe you will pick the one next to the previous one; maybe diagonally opposite.

Now take the board rubber and erase the word that you have written.

Now take the chalk and write, in the middle of the board, the number 2.

Will you make your number straight at the bottom, or loopy?

Now take the rubber and erase the number 2.

Now take the chalk and write the word *sleep* in the corner.

I wonder which corner you chose this time.

Focus on the *e*s as you write. Do you write them separately or loop them together?

Now take the rubber and erase the word *sleep*.

Take your chalk and write, in the centre of the board, the number 3.

How will you write your number 3?

Will you write two equal half circles or will they differ in size?

Now take your rubber and erase the number 3.

Take your chalk and write, in the centre of the board, the number 4.

Is the cross in the number 4 straight up and down? Or does it tilt?

Are the lines straight or curved?

Take your rubber and rub out the number 4.

Now write the word *sleep* in the corner ...

Continue this exercise for as long as it takes, asking similar questions and making observations. You will soon find yourself losing track of the numbers, less able to concentrate on the details. This exercise is extremely effective. Chrissie uses it on a nightly basis and rarely gets beyond the number 6.

V4: Change the sub-modalities

Specific issues	A B C E F S
Gap analysis	7 13 19 20

This visualization exercise will help you to change your perception of pain and traumatic experiences. This technique is specifically to help you manage your noxious symptoms in the here and now. We must acknowledge that, at some point, all traumatic events need to be fully processed.

Take your awareness to your breathing as you have done before.

Allow those breaths to slow and deepen.

Now begin to allow that out breath to become just a little longer than the in breath.

Become aware of the feeling of calm that settles over you.

Now become aware of your pain.

Do not resist it.

Sit in the centre of it, just for the moment.

Become familiar with that old sensation just as it is.

What colour is it?

If you cannot see it, if it had a colour, what colour would it be?

Picture it as clearly as you can.

What shape is it?

Or, if it had a shape, what would it be?

What texture is it?

Is it soft or hard?

Is it smooth or rough?

Now, if your pain made a sound, what would that sound be?

High-pitched or low?

Quiet or loud?

Now, first take your imaginary hands and squash your pain until it is a manageable size.

Good.

Now choose a better colour for your pain.

A favourite colour.

Maybe a calming colour.

Now change the shape of your pain with your imaginary hands.

It is pliable.

Be creative.

Now change its texture in the same way.

Use the tools that you have to make it different from what it was before.

And now change the sound.

Use your memory to choose the sweetest note or happiest sound that you can find and replace the old with the new.

And sit with the new sensation.

V5: Cord cutting in relationships

Specific issues	D F H N
Gap analysis	4 11 12 13 16 17 18

When we form emotional attachments to people, we are bound to them. This means that the behaviour of another person has the power to affect us, either positively or negatively. If this is a detriment to us, we can detach with gratitude and compassion and reclaim that power.

The following exercise will help you to detach from relationships which no longer serve you.

Take your awareness to your breathing.

The tidal in and out of your breath.

As you do this, begin to allow that breath to slow and deepen.

Deeply and slowly.

Become aware of the feeling of calm that settles over you.

It is said that each time we meet someone, a thread is dropped connecting them to us and us to them.

When we meet them again, another is dropped between us.

And again, and again, and again.

Until we know the person well.

And a great cord has been woven from all the threads of all our interactions.

Every interaction weaves a new thread.

Twisting and winding.

And, each time we meet, our conversation is coloured by the presence of the woven cord of our past meetings.

Some cords are masterpieces of design.

Every thread is carefully woven into neat patterns and rows.

And some cords are messy.

With the wiry threads and knots of misunderstanding sticking out of them.

Some cords we would like to keep just as they are.

With some of them, we would like to start again.

To cut the cord and begin with new threads.

Some no longer serve us at all.

Those we would like to cut for good.

Now picture yourself in the centre of a large sphere.

From the centre of this sphere, you can see a great many different cords connecting you with everyone in your life.

How do they appear to you?

Are they neat and organized?

Or messy and chaotic?

Can you see any particular cords that need attention?

Are any of them tangled together?

Sit with how this makes you feel.

Collect this information.

Now, begin with the one cord that most urgently needs work.

Use the tools that you have brought with you.

They are perfect for the job.

Take the cord and ask yourself:

'Do I wish to cut this cord?'

If the answer is 'yes', you can begin.

As you cut the cord, say with your inner voice:

'I release any connections and attachments between us.'

'You are free to go and follow your path in peace.'

'And I am free to follow mine.'

'I wish you well.'

If the answer is 'no' and you find that you are reluctant to cut the cord, it may be that the relationship is ongoing but past experiences and misunderstandings may have distorted your view of each other.

You can either work towards cutting the cord and set an intention to begin afresh.

Or you can work out the tangles and knots to get a clearer picture.

You can then come back at a later date.

Do whatever feels right.

If you cut these cords, you can say:

'I release any past misunderstandings and difficulties that have affected our connection.'

'I set the intention to begin again with new light.'

Each time you set yourself free, visualize a happy future for the person from whom you have detached and wish them well.

V6: Cord cutting for life roles

Specific issues	A B D F G J L M N S
Gap analysis	4 7 12 13 16 17 19

In life we have accepted many roles and labels, all of which restrict us in some way.

The following exercise will help you to detach from your roles and labels so that you can connect with the true authentic part of the Self. This allows you to move forward without restriction, to reach your full potential.

Take your awareness to your breathing.

The tidal in and out of your breath.

As you do this, begin to allow that breath to slow and deepen.

Deeply and slowly.

Become aware of the feeling of calm that settles over you.

Picture yourself in the centre of a large sphere.

Invisible threads connect us to every role and label we have accepted during our time on earth.

This includes personality traits and characteristics.

Some of these will appear as tiny fragile threads, and some as thick, tightly woven ropes.

Depending on the strength and complexity of your attachment to them.

Begin with your gender identity.

Then your name.

Are you someone's child?

Are you a sibling?

A mother or father?

A niece/nephew/aunt/uncle?

Are you someone's friend?

Lover?

What is your title?

What job do you do?

Healer? Lawyer? Advocate? Shopkeeper? Entertainer? Add your own here.

Are you someone's boss?

Employee?

What roles do you play during leisure time?

What additional roles do you play within the family?

Chef? Helper with homework? DIY expert? Wiper of tears? Fetcher of shopping?

What other roles do you play?

Patient? Sufferer? Victim? Addict?

What characteristics have you accepted into your personality?

Are you 'the funny one', 'the clever one', 'the organized one', 'the extrovert', 'the worrier'?

How do you describe yourself?

Picture the cords that connect you to these roles and labels.

Understand that they are *only* roles and labels that you have *chosen* to take up.

Perhaps they have helped you to affirm the approved version of yourself.

They are not who you are.

This is your opportunity to do some pruning.

You can choose to cut no cords at all.

You can cut all of these cords and begin again.

Begin with the cord that most urgently needs attention.

What message do you take from this?

Ask yourself:

'Do I want to cut this cord?'

Listen to the answer.

If you decide to cut the cord, you can begin again.

You can *redefine* that role.

If you want to.

As you cut, say with your inner voice:

'I recognize the role that I have been playing up to now.'

'I know that this role is not who I am.'

'I release my attachment to it so that I may discover my true authentic self.'

'From there I can *choose* which roles I wish to fulfil, and which no longer fit for me.'

Remember that you chose those roles for all the right reasons at the time.

Release them back to their source with kindness and compassion.

V7: Cord cutting for situations

Specific issues	J K O S T
Gap analysis	3 5 6 7 18

When we form emotional attachments to the outcome of situations, we are bound to them. This means that whatever happens with them will have some effect on us. In effect, they have power within our lives. When we detach with gratitude and compassion, we reclaim that power.

The following exercise will help you to detach from situations in your life which no longer serve you.

You may wish to detach from a difficult situation or the outcome of a situation that you are invested in – for example, if you are trying to sell your house, pass an exam or resolve a dispute.

Take your awareness to your breathing.

The tidal in and out of your breath.

As you do this, begin to allow that breath to slow and deepen. Deeply and slowly.

Become aware of the feeling of calm that settles over you.

In every situation, invisible threads connect us to the outcome.

Picture yourself in the centre of a large sphere.

From the centre of this sphere, you can see a great many different cords connecting you with every facet of the situation in question.

In doing this, you will be able to see to which potential outcomes you have a strong emotional attachment.

You may pick this up as a lurching of the stomach or a tightening in the shoulders or chest. It may present as a feeling of excitement or even dread.

It is difficult for a desired outcome to become manifest if we are emotionally attached to it.

Begin with the cord that needs most urgent attention.

As you cut it, say with your inner voice:

'I have taken all action possible to secure a positive outcome.'

'I clearly visualize the desired outcome to this situation.'

'I now release this situation into the universe for the outcome to become manifest.'

Hold the vision of the result as if it already exists.

It is done.

It no longer needs your attention.

V8: Five-finger exercise

Specific issues	A B C D F H R S
Gap analysis	2 15 16 17 19 20

Adapted from David Cheek's original exercise.[2]

This tool is a way to quickly achieve a state of relaxation while, at the same time affirming self-worth. It is very short and simple, and incredibly pleasant to do.

Use it at times in the day when you need a mood boost, or weave it into your self-care ritual to improve self-esteem.

Touch your thumb to your index finger ... As you do so, go back to a time when your body felt healthy fatigue ... Perhaps you had just engaged in an exhilarating physical activity.

Touch your thumb to your middle finger ... As you do so, go back to a time when you had a loving experience. It may be sexual ... It may be a warm embrace ... Or an intimate conversation.

Touch your thumb to your ring finger ... As you do so, go back to the best compliment you have ever received. Try to really accept it now. By accepting it, you are showing high regard for the person who said it. You are really paying him or her a compliment.

Touch your thumb to your little finger ... As you do so, go back to the most beautiful place you have ever been. Stay there for a while, absorbing its beauty.

V9: Fractional induction technique for relaxation

Specific issues	A C E I S
Gap analysis	5 7

To induce physical relaxation, many sources teach the technique of 'tensing and relaxing', but it has been suggested, in physiotherapy teaching, that this may actually lead to an increased tension in our muscles. We prefer the following method of 'fractional induction' which is used in hypnotherapy, where the emphasis for producing the 'relaxation response' is on language and visualization.

Use this meditative exercise to release the physical tension in the body which, in turn, eases turmoil in the brain. It is a great way to get to sleep, but you can do it at any time of the day as a ritual or if you feel that you need it.

Find a quiet, comfortable place.

Begin by bringing your awareness to your breathing.

The tidal in and out of your breath.

Now take three very deep breaths.

Slow and deep.

Follow the air right to the bottom of your lungs, and beyond.

Right to the ends of your fingers.

And the tips of your toes.

As you release the breath, allow any tension that you immediately feel in your body to be released.

And the air fills your body, visualize white light flooding in on the in breath.

And any sources of tension and conflict draining away on the out breath.

Now take your attention to your toes.

Notice any tension that is there and allow it to release, so that they are loose and limp, *just like a hand full of elastic bands.*

Now move your attention to the calves.

Again, allow any tension in the calves to release.

Turning them loose and limp, *just like a handful of elastic bands.*

Opening up all the joints in the feet.

And ankles.

And knees.

Allow this beautiful wave of relaxation to move slowly up the body, paying attention to every muscle.

Every joint.

Slowly and purposefully releasing the tension.

Moving steadily upwards.

Thighs.

Buttocks.

Abdominal muscles.

The broad muscles of the back.

The muscles around the ribcage.

Hands.

Arms.

Shoulders.

Neck and face.

Pay particular attention around the neck and shoulders to really make sure that the tension is fully released.

What are you holding on to?

That needs to be let go.

Continue to breathe slowly and deeply throughout the exercise.

Now, in a deep state of relaxation, focus on your breathing.

In and out.

Slow and deep.

Every time you do this it becomes easier.

And easier.

To relax.

You can stay in this beautifully relaxed state for as long as you need.

When you are ready, slowly bring yourself back to the present situation.

Now, agree to be *kind* to yourself today as you give yourself plenty of time to return to full awareness.

V10: Gather your inner strength

| Specific issues | B D O R S T |
| Gap analysis | 5 7 13 14 15 16 17 18 20 |

Use this tool to bolster your strength so that you are ready for action and can cope with anything. You can also use it to lift your mood.

Find a quiet, comfortable spot.

Take your attention to your breathing.

The tidal in and out of your breath.

Feel the air enter your body.

Bringing life.

Now take your attention to your feet.

Feel the ground beneath them.

Imagine roots spreading down, connecting you to the nutrient-rich earth.

The solid foundation on which everything is built.

Your rock.

Your stability.

Infinite possibilities lying dormant, waiting.

Now take your attention to the top of your head.

Imagine a silver thread connecting you to the cosmos.

The universal source of divine energy.

Visualize the heavens with all their celestial light.

Pure unbounded potential.

Rooted to the earth.

Connected to the universe.

Feel the energy flowing through you.

Now focus on your innermost core.

Do you feel this in your gut, or in your head, or in your heart?

You will know what is right for you.

Feel the energy at your core pulsing.

Your source.

Now feel that energy at your centre start to expand.

Drawing from the earth and the universe.

Feel it gather and multiply.

Feel it grow.

Like a spark that grows to an inferno.

Brighter and brighter.

Warmer and warmer.

Feel your power radiate out until it covers your whole body.

You are infinite energy.

Infinite possibility.

Bask in this feeling for as long as you need.

When you are ready, bring yourself back to full awareness with the knowledge that your inner strength is ready for anything.

V11: Harness the power of your talismans

Specific issues	A B C D H O R T
Gap analysis	5 6 14 15 20

When we believe that an object will bring us power, we imbue it with that power.

In the classic story of Dumbo, the Flying Elephant, *Dumbo finds himself high up on a ledge. The only options available to him are to fall or to fly. Although he does not believe that he can fly, he remembers that he has been given a magic feather which will help him to do just that and, in a leap of faith, he launches into the air. Dumbo knows that, while he has the feather, he can fly. Of course, we learn later on in the story, when Dumbo drops the feather, that he had the power all along. It was his gift, but only in accepting the feather did he give himself permission to use it.*

When using a talisman, we must remember that the gifts it offers already belong to us. In consciously choosing an object and carrying it with us, we are unlocking its power and giving ourselves permission to accept those gifts.

Whatever our objects of significance, the importance lies in the meaning we give them. Equally important are our intentions in using them. Without these, an object is just that.

When we make our power objects conscious, we allow ourselves to receive gifts.

Use this tool whenever you need courage, power, connection, protection, improved performance or healing.

Choose one object that has positive significance for you.

You can do this many times, so do not worry too much about picking the right one.

Sit with your hands on the object.

Think about the reasons why you chose this object.

Does it have specific meaning?

Does it have connections to a specific person or situation?

Is it thought to have healing properties or special powers?

Set clear intentions for the *purpose* of your talisman.

This might be courage, luck, power, protection, improved performance or healing.

Begin to really *connect* with your object of choice.

Allow all the positive emotions and memories that you have concerning this object to come right into the present moment.

Experience them vividly.

What do they look like?

Where do you feel them in your body?

Feel all the power that this object has to offer you.

Allow it to surround you.

Turn up the intensity.

Take your hands off the object and place them in your lap.

Sit with that power.

Know that it is your gift.

Give yourself permission to receive it.

It is yours to use, whenever you need it.

Whether you have your object close at hand or not.

V12: Ideal future visualization

SUPERTOOL

Specific issues	A–T
Gap analysis	1–20

Before we set out on any journey, we must be clear about our destination; we need to be able to see where we are going. To activate the Universal Law of Attraction, we must align with our desired future. To do this we need to be able to visualize it clearly.

This ideal future visualization is a brilliant way to manifest any preferred outcome and is therefore a universal tool. You literally see your desired outcome and the steps you need to take to get to it.

Find a quiet, comfortable spot.

Take your awareness to your breathing.

The tidal in and out of your breath.

Allow your shoulders to soften and fall.

Feel the tension leave your body.

Now, having set a clear intention.

You know what you want to achieve.

See your desired outcome in all its glory.

Hear the cheers and accolades.

Feel the intense satisfaction that comes from accomplishment.

Smell the sweet smell of success.

Taste the victory of having overcome all obstacles.

Genuinely approve of yourself and your achievements.

Clearly visualize your future self.

Exactly as desired.

Happy.

Healthy.

Free of negative behaviours.

With the exactly the right skillset.

You are fulfilled.

You are accomplished.

How does it feel?

Savour this moment; it belongs to you.

It is yours.

When you are ready, bring yourself back to full awareness with the knowledge that you can achieve whatever you set your mind to.

V13: Manage fear

Specific issues	A E F R S
Gap analysis	2 3 14 15 18

Use this tool at times of uncertainty. In acknowledging fear responses and the behaviour that results from them, we can make them conscious. Sometimes merely bearing witness to our own triggers and behaviours is enough to effect positive change. When we are conscious, we have the power to choose.

We can pause.

The next time you feel a fear response rising within you, rather than resisting.

Sit with it.

How and where do you feel it in your body?

Press *pause* on any automatic thoughts, knee-jerk thoughts which follow those feelings.

Instead, become fully present and conscious.

To help you to do this, breathe deeply and slowly, following the air right to the bottom of your lungs.

Thank that protective part of your psyche for rising to the challenge you are facing.

Gently let it know that you are listening.

Come right into the present moment.

Do not concern yourself with any past or future concerns.

Remember that those things cannot be addressed right now.

Ask yourself: 'Is there any immediate threat?'

'Am I projecting myself into a future which is not determined yet?'

Now you can explore what it was that created those feelings of fear.

You can decide whether they were well founded.

You can decide what is needed.

You can choose to surrender to the uncertainty and be present.

You can consciously decide what it is that you need in this moment.

V14: Mindful observation

Specific issues	A C E R
Gap analysis	2 3 5 20

This is a mindfulness exercise to engage in every day. It is based on the concept that fully engaging our senses brings us into the present and leaves no room for past or future. This exercise involves your vision.

Use this tool to bring you into the present moment to prevent rumination about past or future events.

For this exercise, you need to choose a picture or photograph to observe.

Sit in a quiet, comfortable spot.

Place your chosen object in your line of sight.

Close your eyes and take your attention to your breathing.

The tidal in and out of your breath.

Allow your breaths to slow and deepen.

As you do, recognize the characteristic softening of your muscles.

An easing of tension.

Now open your eyes and look at your chosen picture.

Observe the shapes and colours.

The lines.

Appreciate the beauty portrayed for you.

Look at every part.

What details do you see?

Admire any contrasting elements.

Observe the tones, the highlights and shadows.

As you fully focus your attention on your picture.

All other thoughts are on hold.

Not needed.

Not relevant.

Unable to sabotage your mental wellbeing.

Keep your focus on your picture.

As you sit in this state of mindfulness, fully in the present moment.

Feel your connection to the universe.

An immense energy that you can tap into, when needed.

Sit with this true consciousness for as long as you need.

When you are ready, bring yourself back to the room.

Continue your day with your mind at peace. Notice how much more productive you are after enjoying this exercise.

V15: How to reclaim your energy

Specific issues	B C H N S
Gap analysis	4 5 7 12 13 20

Throughout the day, we either give away our energy or it is taken from us. A feeling of powerlessness is extremely negative; it erodes our ability to cope and undermines our resilience.

Use this adaptation of a shamanic 'power retrieval' to reclaim your energy whenever you need to.

Sit in a quiet, comfortable place with your spine straight.

Take your awareness, as always, to your breathing, the tidal in and out of your breath.

Allow those breaths to slow and deepen as you begin to
notice the physical letting go of tension on the out breath.

Now try to get a sense of your need to recharge.

If you are depleted, where does it express itself in your body?

Does it have a colour?

A taste?

A smell?

What does it *feel* like?

Sit with it for a moment.

Now imagine yourself on a path.

At the beginning of a journey.

This journey represents a recent difficult day.

It represents a journey where you lost some of your energy.

However the path appears is right for you.

No need to question or analyse.

Just accept that this is the path where you can reclaim your
power.

Begin walking.

As you walk along the path, you will notice objects which
have been left along the side of it.

These objects represent your energy.

It doesn't matter what they are, just know that they symbolize
part of your power that you have either lost or given away.

As you travel along the path, pick up these objects and put
them in the bag that you have brought with you.

Continue along, collecting the lost objects, until you know
that you have reached the end of the journey or you arrive
back at the start.

Now sit down in a comfortable spot with your bag.

When you examine the contents, you will notice that the
objects have merged together into a ball of light.

Take out this ball of light. It belongs to you.

Now return it.

You can press it towards your heart or breathe in into your
chest.

However you choose to reclaim the energy is right for you.

Enjoy feeling yourself fill with radiant light as you own that
lost energy once more.

Sit for a few more moments and then begin to drift gently
back to full awareness, with a replenished zest for life and
the resilience to face everything that lies ahead.

V16: Sleep induction technique

Specific Issues	A I R
Gap Analysis	3 7

*This technique is adapted from a hypnotherapy induction script devised
by Terence Watts.[3] It is based on the neurological concept that people can
hold only between five and nine conscious thoughts in their short-term
memory.[4] Encouraging people to concentrate on more than nine things
overloads this, and they can be more easily led into trance.*

Use this tool here, with the end goal being sleep.

Make yourself comfortable in bed.

Follow each of these instructions very slowly.

The aim of the exercise is to bring your awareness to a new
and different sensation or thought, changing it at regular,
slow intervals.

The order of each thought or change in awareness is not
important.

It does not matter if you repeat certain changes of awareness
or add in your own.

The key is to keep slowly and repetitively bringing your
awareness to something different until your conscious mind
becomes overloaded and gives way to an altered state.

Once you are deeply relaxed, sleep will follow ...

Place your right hand on your stomach and your left hand
on your chest.

Take deep, regular breaths in.

Feel your right hand rise and your left hand stay steady as
you breathe deeply into your stomach.

Feel the pillow underneath your head.

How soft it is.

And the way your head presses deeply into its softness.

Smell the familiar smells of your bedroom.

Or any aromatherapy oils you have added to your pillow.

Feel the indent in the mattress on your bed.

From the pressure of your body as gravity pulls you deeper
and deeper in.

Listen to the sound of silence in your room.

There is never complete silence.

Recognize the comforting sounds inside and outside your
home.

Feel the warmth of your body.

As it relaxes into the bed.

Surrounding you.

Drawing you deeper and deeper into a state of relaxation.

Listen to the quiet, regular sound of your heartbeat.

That is always there, but not noticed in our busy days.

Feel the air filling your lungs.

Deeper and deeper.

Feel the pressure of the covers pressing into your body.

Keeping you.

Cocooning you.

Making you safe and secure.

Feel yourself pulled deeper and deeper.

Into the realms of sleep.

Where your body will repair itself.

Making you healthier and stronger.

Ready for a healthy, vibrant tomorrow.

21

Practical exercises

P1: Assertiveness techniques

Specific issues	A D G N P
Gap analysis	1 8 11 12 16 17 18 19 20

There is a big difference between assertiveness and aggression. The most assertive demeanour is to be silent, listen and answer appropriately. Assertiveness is stating your truth. Stick to facts and keep emotion out of it.

Follow the guide below when you want to be more assertive.

1. Listen with kindness and attention to others' point of view. Come at everything from a position of respect.
2. Use 'I' statements when you want to take responsibility for the content, including saying how you feel about what has happened.
3. Think about the words you are using:
   - Regarding your intentions: I could → I will and I have to → I choose to
   - In requests: Could you just ...? or Do you mind doing xyz ...? → Please do xyz
4. Give yourself time. If a request comes, don't jump to answer; thank the person for the information and give them a time frame for your reply.
5. Script your reply. State the event/situation, explain your feelings, state what you want and relay positive expected outcomes.

6. Value yourself and your rights and voice your point of view confidently. Maintain your message – prepare it and keep restating it. Keep your tone and pitch calm.
7. Escalation – politely and respectfully escalate through consequences and hierarchical layers.
8. Acknowledge you cannot control the behaviour of others.
9. Be positive in your communication – verbal and non-verbal – and open in your body language.
10. Be open to feedback but avoid apologizing for things you are not responsible for.

P2: Compartmentalization exercises

Specific issues	A B C F H N O S
Gap analysis	1 2 3 8 9 10 15 19 20

Use this organizational exercise to help compartmentalize what is happening in your life, work, your feelings and past trauma.

Compartmentalizing tasks

Start by separating your thoughts into channels that represent all the things that are happening in your life right now. You can label these – for example 'Work' 'Family', 'Studies' 'Current crises'.

To create these separate compartments, you can visualize them in different ways. As a filing cabinet with different drawers. Auditory people may separate the streams by recognizing different voices; your own voice with different styles that represent the contents of your compartment. Kinaesthetic people may want to actually have different drawers and put something that represents their compartments in each. Use different colours or sounds. Your unconscious mind knows how best to perceive this. However it appears is right for you. Imagine if you spoke only Spanish at home and English at work. How much easier would it be to switch cleanly from one compartment to another?

- Allot time for each compartment and set boundaries. For example 6.30 to 7.30am is me time; from 7.30 to 8.30am make sure everyone is ready, for school and work.
- Clearly transition between compartments and have a way of doing this – visualize closing the drawer on one work stream and opening the next. Tune out one voice so another comes to the fore. Put one object in its box and get out the next. Again, set boundaries – for example, on the way home give yourself a time frame to reflect on the day and process what happened, but, at the last traffic light before home, stop thinking about work – put that away and start thinking about home.
- Consider when your peak performance times are and plan your day accordingly.
- Don't multitask. This discourages compartmentalization and doesn't support your separate streams.
- When you are in each compartment, give that area all your attention. Listen 100 per cent to what you are doing – *be present*. Turn off your phone so you have no distractions.
- If things pop into your head while you are focused on one task, rather than trying to keep them in your head, jot them down so you don't forget later, then push them out of your consciousness.

Compartmentalizing emotions and trauma

This is a *short-term tool* to alleviate suffering. Remember that *all* traumas must be processed. If you are compartmentalizing, you are doing it to get through a certain situation or time. To move forward you must unpack what has happened and process it. Put time aside to do this. The core skills and other tools in this section will help.

To help you through difficult situations in the short term, try the following:

- Allocate a set amount of time – 'I will give myself one hour and then write down everything that I think and feel about the situation,' or talk about it for a set amount of time and then it is time to stop. You haven't necessarily dealt with the pain but you won't let it ruin your day.
- Remember your compartments are there – you can go in at any time – so move away from thinking you have to deal with and process every crisis that happens immediately.
- Ground yourself and remind yourself to be present. Remember to only address what is in front of you right now. Ask: 'Is thinking/dwelling/ruminating on this going to change anything? Am I moving forward here or just going round in circles?' If the answer is 'circles', then you need to recognize the limitations of the situation and focus on what you can change, thinking more in terms of solutions.
- Ask, 'How much more productive would I be if I wasn't thinking about this right now?' If the answer is 'much more', then stop and get on with what you are supposed to be doing.

P3: Delegating

Specific issues	C N O P
Gap analysis	1 5 6 8 9 10 11

Good leadership is about recognizing the person best suited to do a task. We often don't delegate as we feel we are offloading work. Sometimes we think we can do the task better. Delegating can also help us when our workload feels overwhelming.

Follow the steps below and start to delegate effectively, reducing your task burden.

1. Prepare yourself to delegate by letting go of ego. Recognize the benefits of delegating and don't wait for a volunteer.
2. Rate tasks by effort level and skill level required and delegate high-effort, low-skill tasks.
3. Know your team and their capabilities. Delegate to the appropriate person.
4. Give clear instructions and clear outcomes with the task – that is, be clear about your intentions.
5. Be prepared to teach people new skills and allocate them enough resources.
6. Trust but verify. This means check they are on task at various points, but allow them the freedom to create the desired outcome in their own way.
7. Feedback – this is a two-way process. Say 'thank you'. We are often quick to pick on things that people do that annoys us, so we should take time to pass on praise as well.

A great exercise is to log all the tasks you have completed in a day. When you have the list of tasks, think about who else currently in your team *could* have done each task.

Also think about who else might have been able to do it (even if they don't currently work with you). Looking at the list you may well see opportunities to reorganize your workload and create ideas for new roles.

P4: Develop an internal locus of control

Specific issues	D O Q R
Gap analysis	2 3 6 14 15 18

To stay afloat on rough seas, it is imperative that we address our 'locus of control'. Believing that we can influence what happens via our responses makes us highly resilient.

To move your locus of control towards the internal end of the spectrum:

1. Be aware of what you can and cannot control. Factors you cannot control are your limitations, and energy spent trying to change them is wasted.
2. Recognize that you are fully in control of all of your thoughts, feelings and behaviours. No one has the power to affect your emotions unless you choose to let them.
   - If someone is rude, they are rude.
   - *You* decide how to respond.
   - You can even choose whether it affects you or not.
   - No one has the power to make you angry, upset or confrontational unless you give that power to them.
   - Take responsibility for all your responses.
3. Reframe negative responses. When you notice a negative response in yourself – it may be physical (e.g. a sick feeling in your stomach, a tight chest or palpitations) or a thought ('I'm not good enough', 'I have failed') – stop and take a moment to examine that response. Ask yourself:
   - Why has this response been triggered?
   - Is my response appropriate?
   - Is my response helpful?
   - Is there a different response that would be more appropriate or more useful?

P5: Eisenhower's time management tool

Specific issues	O
Gap analysis	1 8 9 10

Time is a valuable asset and is the only thing we cannot get back. Eisenhower's principle of time management is a useful, practical tool to help you stay in control of your day-to-day tasks and your long-term goals.

Dwight Eisenhower was the 34th president of the United States. He was, before that, an officer in the US military. In both these roles he had to make big decisions, and so he developed a matrix to help. Stephen Covey uses this principle as an example of good practice in his book *The 7 Habits of Highly Effective People*.[1]

Tasks can be categorized in terms of their importance and their urgency:

	URGENT	NOT URGENT
IMPORTANT	DO IT	PLAN IT
NOT IMPORTANT	DELEGATE IT	DUMP IT

Get into the habit of categorizing your tasks regularly. This can be part of setting your intentions for the day:

- *Do* the important and urgent ones first, regardless.
- *Plan* the important, non-urgent ones into your diary.
- *Delegate* the important, non-urgent ones.
- *Dump* the rest.

P6: Five-point rescue plan

SUPERTOOL

Specific issues	A–T
Gap analysis	1–20

This is a strategic, problem-solving framework to help you sort through any situation. As it is so versatile, it is a universal tool.

The key to creating a 'five-point rescue plan' is to accurately identify the problem. All too often we concentrate on the symptoms we experience, attempting to alleviate them, rather than addressing their true cause.

Ask yourself the following questions:

1. Why am I stuck?
2. Did something happen beyond my control?
3. What are my limitations?

4. What stops me from moving forward?
5. Who affects my situation?

Using your answers, fill out the table below – sorting through the thoughts, feelings and behaviours involved in your situation.

What is my perceived problem?	Examples: *I am worried about coronavirus* *I am in pain* *I am overweight.*
What are my negative behaviours?	Examples: *Ruminating about things out of my control* *Giving attention to my pain* *Overeating*
What drives these behaviours?	Examples: *Fear, anger, apathy, boredom, guilt, ego*
What are my limitations?	Examples: *A diagnosis* *The behaviour of others* *Finances*
What can I change?	Examples: *What I think, feel and do*
What is my actual problem?	Examples: *Lack of purpose* *Lack of self-esteem* *Communication problems*

Look at your table:

- Accept your limitations – you cannot change them.
- Focus on the actual problem you have identified and concentrate on the things you can change.

It is important to remember that making massive changes is neither practical nor sustainable. Radical changes in habit are hard to maintain because they are unfamiliar to us. They may be relatively easy to apply at first, while the motivation to change is at its greatest but, if success is not achieved quickly, we often revert back to our previous, more comfortable habits.

Choose five small but significant changes you can make to your life and do them every day.

My five-point rescue plan

1.
2.
3.
4.
5.

Implement your plan, weaving the changes into your day.

Evaluate the response. If it isn't working, change your points or check you are looking at the right problem. You may also be blocking progress because of fear. This is thoroughly discussed in Chapters 6 and 8.

P7: Gratitude journal

SUPERTOOL

Specific issues	A–T
Gap analysis	1–20

A grateful mind-set is a prerequisite to resilience. Use this tool to help you to live gratefully and attract abundance. This is a universal concept and so the tool will apply to any situation.

Below is a framework for creating a gratitude journal:

Make time in your bedtime routine for gratitude.

Turn off devices.

Find a comfortable place to sit, surrounded by things you love. This may be outside; it may be in your bedroom. Wherever feels right for you.

Make sure you have no distractions.

Prepare yourself for your journalling by centring yourself.

Close your eyes and take your awareness, as always, to your breathing.

Feel the ground beneath your feet, the cushions behind you or the chair against your legs.

Listen carefully to the sounds around you.

Breathe deeply and slowly.

Feel your connection to the universe.

Now open your eyes and start to write:

Think about three things you are grateful for today.

How do they make you feel?

Sit with that feeling, relive it.

Even on bad days there are positive elements. Focus on these.

Now think about the things you have achieved today and write about them.

Congratulate yourself.

Give yourself permission to feel proud.

Write down three things you have learned today.

Feel grateful for those lessons.

In the silence, allow your intentions for tomorrow to crystallize.

Clear intentions lead to positive outcomes.

P8: Habit analysis form

Specific issues	G J L M N Q
Gap analysis	1 2 4 6 7 8 9 10

This form can be used to identify the losses and gains that relate to your habit. The habit that you are addressing could be alcohol, cigarettes or even a repetitive, negative behaviour such as overeating. You may see the symptoms of your habit first. It is important to recognize their cause and identify the nature of your habit.

For example, damage to relationships at home due to not being present may be down to your timekeeping habits, your addiction to your status at work, or repetitive worries about whether you have done a good enough job.

By examining the various costs of your habit, you can outline factors which will motivate you to make positive changes. By addressing the benefits and gains, you will be able to identify your attachments to the habit.

Listing alternatives will allow you to explore ways to replace the negative behaviour with something that serves you better.

To affect this change, you can follow this up with a 'six-step reframe', a 'five-point rescue plan', thought diaries, gratitude journals, and meditations for detachment and cleansing.

Use the following table as the basis for creating your own habit analysis form.

How does my habit affect my relationships?	
How does my habit affect my mental health?	
How does my habit affect my physical health?	
How does my habit affect my career?	
How does my habit affect my finances?	
What am I gaining from this habit?	
What can I do differently?	

P9: How to say 'no'

Specific issues	D N O P
Gap analysis	1 5 8 9 10 12

Saying 'yes' is easy but, if this leads to more work than you can manage, no one wins.

Use this tool to help you develop the skills and confidence to say 'no' without creating an issue. Remember that we need to set clear intentions and, when we do, all our communications, both verbal and non-verbal, will be aligned.

Make your responses conscious rather than automatic. Remember that a habitual need to say 'yes' may be a result of your conditioning, core beliefs, shadow and archetypes. You may wish to explore this using the theory section of this book (Part 1). In the meantime, here is a practical tool.

Before answering any request, give yourself time to consider it:

- What is the commitment?
- How strongly do you feel about the project?
- Is the request in your job description?

Do not say 'yes' out of a sense of obligation or of guilt about saying 'no'. Guilt is a destructive emotion that will generate bad feeling. Saying 'no' for the right reasons is the right thing to do.

It is OK to say 'no'. If you don't have the time or inclination for the job, you are not the best person for it and it is better to say this.

When you decide to say 'no', do not give an explanation as to why. This provokes the other party to problem-solve for you and opens up a discussion about how to change your mind. Just say 'no' calmly and with respect.

P10: Making connections

Specific issues	A B C D H N P T
Gap analysis	11 12 16 17 18

We are breathing the same air as every other living thing. We are living under the same sunshine and moonlight, and are nourished and sustained by the same earth.

Use these exercises to improve your connections with others, with nature and with Self.

Here are some practical things to do:
Connect with those who share your home:

- Make time to talk.
- Suggest fun activities that you can do together.
- Enlist help with completing useful tasks.
- Share your thoughts and offer support to those you live with.

Check in with family, friends, colleagues and neighbours via:

- phone
- virtual platform
- letter
- over the fence (at an appropriate distance).

Connect with nature:

- Enjoy a walking meditation.
- Exercise outdoors.
- Tend to some seedlings or plants.
- Play with your pets.

Connect to Self:

- Consider your purpose. What is it that you want to do in this life?
- Write a list of your qualities and achievements.
- Make time to do one leisure activity that you enjoy every day.
- Create something.
- Make your home a place which reflects your tastes and interests.

Highly ascended spiritual masters spend much time alone but do not suffer from symptoms of isolation. This is because they understand wider connection.

Aspire to be content when in your own company, in the knowledge that you are never alone.

P11: Motivational tool

Specific issues	B D J O
Gap analysis	7 9 10

Motivation is vital. Often, we know what we need to do and what we should do, but we can't get started. This then leads to negative thoughts about 'not being good enough, affirming negative core beliefs which, in turn, promote apathy.

Use this tool to kick-start your motivation.

Set clear intentions

What do you want to achieve? This will help you focus and trigger your motivation. Without a clear intention, we manifest chaos and can quickly feel overwhelmed. You may have experienced this when your to-do list is so long, or the house is so untidy, that you do not know where to start.

Plan

How will you do it? Make the first step small and achievable – even if this means splitting tasks down into micro-tasks. Make sure you have the right equipment and enough time for your tasks. We can become demotivated if we don't.

Undertake the first step

Start. Really push yourself here; you have to start. This is why it is useful to make the first step very small. Set a date and start; no matter what it is and however small, starting will get you going, and, once you start, you will be more motivated to continue.

Review regularly

Monitoring your progress and giving positive feedback keeps us motivated and on track. If things are going well, that is great. If they are not, give yourself a break and go back to your intentions. Check your plan. It is important to acknowledge any bumps along the journey but don't let them stop you moving forward.

P12: NLP during conflict

Specific issues	D E G N O P R
Gap analysis	11 12 13 19 20

Use this tool during a conflict situation. It will allow you to step back from any emotions caused by the altercation and speak your truth with respect.

When you are faced with a conflict situation, press *pause*:

1. Become aware of your internal responses. Allow yourself to step into the shoes of your Observer Self. This means stepping back from any emotions that have arisen because of the conflict. Notice what has provoked you and allow yourself to be grateful for the information. Accept that your internal response is about *you* and not them.
2. Slow down your breathing and responses to create gaps within the conversation. This allows you to manage the pace of the interaction. It facilitates processing of information and allows you to give conscious responses rather than reacting to what triggered you.
3. Remember to use the Thank You Technique. Say with sincerity, 'Thank you for your comments', remembering that you are thanking the universe for the opportunity to examine why what was said provoked you so much.
4. When unsure how to respond, create a space. Long, tangible pauses in a conversation are extremely powerful when *you* have created them. Any discomfort they create is felt only by the other party. You can then follow with something like 'Here's how I would like to respond to that.'
5. Come at everything from a position of respect.

P13: Observe your locus of power

Specific issues	N P T
Gap analysis	4 11 12 19 20

We can improve our resilience by observing our own behaviour in all our communications. Collecting information like this allows us to spot patterns and, eventually, make our responses conscious rather than unconscious. This tool is a step-by-step guide through this process.

Use this tool during communication and conflict.

Spend some time observing your own behaviour during conversations, in all areas of your life. Do this with kindness towards yourself and others. Remember that the purpose of this exercise is to improve your understanding of Self.

See whether you can spot patterns. You may like to write down transcripts of conversations after they have happened and decide the position of the locus of power. You do not need to take any further action at this stage. Sometimes simply raising your awareness of power dynamics alone, can effect positive change.

If you want to, you can then pause and ask yourself the following questions:

- 'What am I seeking from this person by saying this?'
- 'Is this something that I can give to myself?'

You can then ask:

- 'What is this telling me about what my needs are in terms of developing resilience?'

This will show you where you need to work. Here, you can explore your own need for approval/permission/reassurance etc.

Some examples:

- Are you constantly seeking approval?
- Do you regularly need permission to go ahead with projects?

- Are you running everything by someone else so that you do not have to take responsibility when things go wrong?
- Do you regularly communicate your talents and achievements?
- Do you compete with your peers?
- Do you enjoy gossip?
- What do you seek to gain from each interaction?
- Can you give these things to yourself so that you do not need them from others?
- Can you take more responsibility when interacting with others?

There are many reasons why we might shift the locus of power towards others and, therefore, away from the Self. Exploring the reasons why you interact in the way that you do will improve your understanding and lead to more conscious communication.

Power dynamics are complex. There will always be both a balance and an exchange of power in human interaction. Sometimes, we must give away some of our power for a useful interaction to take place. The key is to raise our awareness and consciously choose what is appropriate, rather than acting out of unconscious need.

Understanding and mastering our part in the 'great dance' of communication is both enlightening and empowering. In fact, it is key to building resilience and staying afloat in modern times.

P14: Organization – prioritization and efficiency

Specific issues	C O
Gap analysis	1 8 9 10 12

Use this tool to maximize your efficiency. Remember to set clear intentions.

1. Make a list of all your tasks.
2. The MindTools Action Priority Matrix Worksheet[2] helps you to prioritize tasks. Rate tasks by impact and effort:

- Low-effort, high-impact tasks are 'quick wins'.
- High-effort, low-impact tasks are 'thankless tasks'.

3. Prioritize your tasks accordingly.
4. Do not procrastinate – do it, delegate it or dump it.
5. Delegate jobs appropriately (see P3).
6. Say 'no' when appropriate (see P9).

P15: Reframe core beliefs

Specific issues	D G Q
Gap analysis	3 6 8 16 17 19

Use this tool to help analyse thought patterns and, specifically, identify core beliefs. Negative core beliefs can then be reframed using the table below.

Event	Thoughts and feelings	Cognitive illusions	Underlying core belief	Reframe the belief	New mantra

Catalogue the event. Describe what thoughts were in your head and how you felt. Next, examine the thought – what is the evidence for and against it?

Can you see any obvious cognitive illusions (see Chapter 15)?[3] These include:

- catastrophizing
- jumping to conclusions
- making assumptions
- fortune telling
- mind reading
- selective evidence gathering
- overgeneralizing.

Consider the Universal Law of Reflection. Consider your shadow. What core belief does this pattern of thinking point to?

- I am worthless (inadequate, a failure).
- I am unlovable.
- I am bad.
- I am defective.
- I am different.

In the same way, apply the Socratic questions to this core belief:

1. Is this belief realistic?
2. Am I basing my belief on facts or on emotions?
3. What is the evidence for this belief?
4. Could I be misinterpreting that evidence?
5. Am I viewing the situation as black and white when it's really more complicated?

When the answer to these questions is 'no', you need to reframe the belief to a positive:

- Worthless becomes PRECIOUS.
- Unlovable becomes CHERISHED.
- Defective becomes PERFECT.

Your new mantra is:

- 'I am a precious human being.'
- 'I am cherished.'
- 'I am perfect.'

You need to affirm these new mantras on a daily basis. Say them aloud in the mirror. You have to believe them to be true.

Apply the same Socratic questioning to help affirm these beliefs and keep a 'positive core belief' log.

P16: Reframe fearful thoughts – ATOMS tool

Specific issues	A D E G Q R
Gap analysis	2 3 6 14 15 19

This tool is a great template for reframing fearful thoughts. Use this tool whenever you feel fearful thoughts dictating your feelings and behaviours.

When a fearful thought enters our head, we need to take the time to acknowledge its presence. Ignoring thoughts and trying to push them away or into a box is resistance. This is counter-productive because the thought is still present; we have only pushed it deeper into the psyche. We are not listening, and so we are encouraging it to shout louder.

When we seek to *acknowledge* the thought, we can process it, and then reframe it. Going further than acknowledgment we, in fact, need to *thank* the universe for the thought and indeed the fear from which it stemmed. Everything that happens to us, good or bad, is a lesson. Being grateful for every lesson is walking the path towards positivity.

Next, we need to *observe* the fearful thought. What is it trying to tell us? Where does it come from and what does it want? Observation with emotion is, in fact, overanalysis and this should be avoided. The observation needs to be without the emotions that fuel distorted thinking. *Step back* and observe with compassion, for yourself and any others involved.

Once you can truly see where the fearful thought has come from. Only then can you *measure* its validity. What is the evidence for it and against it? Again, *step back* and do not let emotions cloud your assessment.

When you have observed the validity of your fearful thought, you can *consciously select* your response. Will you repeat the same negative cycle? Or will you move forward in a positive way?

Will you *evolve*? Or will you *repeat*?

A	Acknowledge the thought
T	Thank the universe for the lesson
O	Observe the thought without emotion
M	Measure the validity of the thought
S	Select your response

P17: Self-care assessment

Specific issues	C N O T
Gap analysis	4 5 7 8 12 13 16 17

The first and most important step towards learning to practise Self-care is to know your Self. You can listen to all the recommendations of the vast number of experts in the field of human wellbeing but, without a profound knowledge of the Self, it is impossible to know your own needs. Once these are established, a plan for meeting them can be made.

Use this tool when you feel that your life is out of balance. Better still, get into the habit of using it on a regular basis to keep you on track. This tool works best if used after the Self-check (P18).

Set aside time and ask yourself the following questions. Write down your answers. Do this consciously.

What do I need more of in my life?

This is a limitless list of those things which you may have already identified as sustaining and nourishing you – for example meditation, music, art, dancing, swimming, reading, cinema, theatre, socializing. You may describe them as 'good for the soul', but, unless you are committed to the practice of Self-care, it is unlikely that you will make enough time or space for them in your daily life. Take your time with this, and do not allow any limitations to discourage you. Once you have listed these, you can place them in order of importance.

What do I need less of in my life?

These may be necessary to your job or home life in some way but, with a little help, consideration and planning, could be reduced in number, volume or intensity – for example bills, debts, work, meetings, arguments, chores, accidents, misplaced items. Again, order these in terms of importance. You may wish to record how much of your time is taken up with these activities.

What will I no longer put up with in my life?

This is a full stop. What things are you no longer willing to tolerate? Once you have made this promise to yourself, you must be clear and disciplined with your boundaries so that they are understood and adhered to by all concerned – especially you. No exceptions.

Now, look at your lists of desires and obligations. They have much information to offer you in terms of your Self-care needs.

You can now create your Self-care Plan – for example, looking at ways of managing your time and adjusting your activities to increase the things that nourish you and minimize those that drain you. There are multiple tools in the Resilience Toolkit to help with you with your Self-care Plan.

Self-care is often portrayed as a collection of kind and gentle acts towards the Self which, ultimately, create feelings of wellbeing. However, when we are being kind and gentle towards the Self, it can be all too easy to 'cut ourselves some slack' and give up on our goals. This is resistance. The paradox here is that the goal is Self-care.

One crucial but often overlooked aspect of Self-care is commitment to practice. This takes discipline. It can be difficult to commit to yourself when you have people and projects depending on you and you perceive that the world is watching and judging. *The only thing that matters here is what is going on for you.*

During our years of research, we have found that those who add certain practices into their lives such as meditation, yoga, dietary changes and exercise reap far better rewards when they are committed.

Make a promise to yourself to commit to your Self-care. Be clear and precise. We have often heard it said that 'you cannot pour from an empty cup'. It is time to tend to your Self.

P18: Self-check

Specific issues	A B C R S T
Gap analysis	3 5 7 13 16 17 18 20

This tool is best used ritualistically throughout the day. Asking yourself set questions regarding your wellbeing regularly allows you to identify the appropriate issues to address. This will give you direction for your thought processes and actions and, in turn, improve your day. You can also use this tool when you are feeling overwhelmed.

Choose appropriate small gaps in your day to ask yourself the following questions (e.g. in the car before you go into work, before meetings, comfort breaks, lunch, in the car before you leave or in the car before you enter your house):

1. What do I want to achieve right now?
2. What is taking up most of my thinking right now?
3. What am I feeling right now?
4. What is draining me?
5. What is supporting me?

Now bring yourself back to the present and refocus your energy and your activities.

In generating answers to these questions, you can address any underlying issues which may be drawing your focus away from your current tasks. You can see that, ideally, the answers to the first two questions should be aligned, but, often, our thoughts are distracted away from the present moment by pressing concerns from elsewhere in our lives.

Moving on to tools such as compartmentalization, reframing and mindfulness would be useful here.

P19: Six-step reframe

Specific issues	A B D G J K L M Q R
Gap analysis	2 3 6 7 13 19 20

This NLP exercise is one of the most useful techniques for reframing a behaviour or habit. It is practised in hypnotherapy and psychotherapy intervention. Adapted from Bandler and Grinder.[4]

Sit in a comfortable place where you will not be disturbed. You may wish to keep a pen and paper handy to record your thoughts and emotions for reference and processing.

1. Identify the behaviour that you want to change. Be specific and succinct. Use simple language. Remain emotionally detached. For example, 'I wish to stop eating as a result of becoming upset.'
2. Go to the part of your psyche that is responsible for running this behaviour. Try to get a *sense* of where this is. This part of the exercise requires intuition rather than logical thought.
3. Say either aloud or in your mind:

   - I wish to change the behaviour of [*eating as a result of becoming upset*].
   - This is because this behaviour is outmoded and no longer serves me.
   - I recognize that this behaviour was programmed for all the right reasons at the time and that it has kept me safe up to now. For that, I am grateful.
   - I acknowledge that this is only *one* way to manage the behaviour of [*becoming upset*] and that there are other behaviours which may be more appropriate for me now.
   - I would like to request to try some alternative behaviours for the situation of [*becoming upset*] which are more appropriate to my current circumstances and which suit me better.

   Before you move on, try to get the sense that you have the permission of that part of the psyche to try a new behaviour.
4. Now go to the creative part of your psyche. This is the part with all the ideas and solutions. Explain that you would like it to suggest some alternative behaviour for the situation

(becoming upset) to replace the current one (eating). Pause and allow the creative part of the psyche to come up with suggestions. They may present in different ways. Give yourself time. Do not overthink.

5. Select the alternative behaviours that appeal to you the most and take them to the part of you that ran the original behaviour. Tell that part that you would like it to run one or more of the alternative behaviours that have been suggested for responding to [*becoming upset*] because they are more appropriate to your situation and, therefore, serve you better. Reassure it that any changes can be reversed if the new way of behaving does not appear to be working. Ask that part of the psyche if it is willing to take responsibility for this from now on.

- Wait until you feel that you have a positive response.
- Now take some time to visualize yourself in the future, in the situation of [*becoming upset*].

Now take yourself forward in time by 24 hours. Watch your new behaviours and responses coming into play. Watch the situation play out positively. See that you are safe when you respond in this way. Notice how it feels to have selected a behaviour that serves you well. Take yourself forward one week and do the same. Now fast-forward one month. You can visualize the positive effects of releasing the unwanted behaviour (in our example: weight loss, better body image, improved confidence). By visualizing six months ahead, you see yourself in a whole new light.

6. Now bring all parts of the psyche together. Imagine that you are having a general meeting where every part has a voice. Ask *all* parts whether they are happy for this change to take place. If you get that sense that all parts agree, then the reframe is done. If you sense a lack of agreement, return to step 2 and repeat the process from there, addressing the objection.

P20: Standing tall: a two-minute resilience exercise

Specific issues	A B C D G N O
Gap analysis	2 5 7 18 20

Use this tool ritualistically every day to boost your confidence and make you feel more in control. Spend two minutes per day in an open, 'powerful' stance.

Social scientist Amy Cuddy and her team found that effecting a closed defensive position for two minutes resulted in a 10 per cent decrease in testosterone and an 11 per cent increase in cortisol: lower confidence and higher stress. A confident open pose for two minutes resulted in a 20 per cent increase in testosterone and a 25 per cent decrease in cortisol; higher confidence and lower stress.[5]

Open postures are those with uncrossed arms and legs, shoulders back and head up. Think Wonder Woman and Superman stances!

1. Pick your open pose – the more open the better.
2. Stand tall for two minutes. Focus on your breathing and allow the body chemistry to develop.

Make this exercise a part of your morning ritual. It will have an effect on your brain that makes you feel assertive and relaxed. Listen to Amy's inspirational TED Talk, following the link: <https://www.youtube.com/watch?v=Ks-_Mh1QhMc>

P21: Tips for making the most of your time

Specific issues	C O
Gap analysis	1 8 9 10

In childhood, all experiences are new. As we get older, less so. This explains, in part, why time appears to pass more quickly as we age.

Our emotions, of course, will also have an impact on our perceptions. When we are afraid, time expands. We become stuck and a bad experience can seem to last for ever.

Use this tool to help you to make the most of your time.

- Create new experiences whenever possible. That means trying new things, saying 'yes' and being open to receive what the universe has to offer you. The more memories you have of an event, the more space that event takes up in your psyche and the longer the event appears to have lasted.
- Stay present in all things. If your thoughts are in the past or future, you will not fully experience what is happening now and you certainly will not be creating memories.
- Remember that emotion manipulates perception, so avoid adding unnecessary emotional weight to events, either before or after they have happened. This will prevent wasting time worrying about the future or revisiting the past.
- Limit time on social media/technology.
- Formalize time for connecting with loved ones.
- Set time aside to enjoy nature.
- Banish guilt for time spent on Self-care.

P22: Thought reframe

SUPERTOOL

Specific issues	A–T
Gap analysis	1–20

Thought patterns are evident in every aspect of life, making this a universal tool. Our core beliefs influence our thoughts about every situation; however, we are not at their mercy. We can challenge unhelpful thoughts and choose to think constructively, creating a resilient mind-set.

Use this tool to help analyse your thoughts. You can recognize and challenge unhelpful patterns.

Date	Event	Thought	Feeling	Cognitive illusion	Reframe
Monday	Late for work	I am so useless My boss is going to be mad I might get fired	Nervous, sick stomach Anxious Heart racing	Over-generalization Catastrophizing Mind reading Making assumptions	I am late for work Tomorrow I will pack my bag the night before so I have more time

Catalogue the event. Describe what thoughts were in your head and how you felt. Next, examine the thought – what is the evidence for and against it?

Can you see any obvious cognitive illusions (see Chapter 15)?[6] These include:

- catastrophizing
- jumping to conclusions
- making assumptions
- fortune telling
- mind reading
- selective evidence gathering
- overgeneralizing.

Consider how the Universal Law of Reflection (Chapter 4), your shadow self (Chapter 5) and survival archetypes (Chapter 6) may be influencing the cycle.

Can you think of a different thought that is less damaging?

Reframe your cognitive behavioural cycle. See the Six-step reframe tool (P19). Remember, reframing thoughts is good work but, unless you reframe the underlying core belief, you will be reframing for the rest of your life. See the Reframe core belief tool (P15).

You can catalogue your day in more detail in a classic thought diary or journal, or, indeed, with pictures or music. As discussed in Chapter 15, this exercise has positive benefits for mental health.

If you note any repetitive negative thinking, you can identify from which core belief it arises. You can then use one of the core belief reframe techniques.

P23: Ujjayi breathing

Specific issues	A E F R
Gap analysis	14 15 20

Use this breathing exercise to stimulate the vagal nerve, which activates the parasympathetic system and the relaxation response. It is particularly helpful for panic attacks.

Sit with your spine straight.

Close your eyes.

Take your awareness to your breathing.

Breathe in and out through your nose.

Keep the in breath and out breath an equal length, measured and controlled.

With each breath fill your belly, allowing it to stick out.

As you inhale and exhale, constrict your throat making a rasping noise (a Darth Vader-like sound).

As little as two minutes of Ujjayi breathing is enough to centre your mind and terminate a panic attack.

Notes

Chapter 1

1 Garmezy, N., Stress-resistant children: The search for protective factors. *Recent research in developmental psychopathology*, 4 (1985), 213–33.

2 Werner, E. E., *The Children of Kauai: A Longitudinal Study from the Prenatal Period to Age Ten.* University of Hawaii Press, Honolulu, 1971.

3 Adler, A., *The Practice and Theory of Individual Psychology.* Martino Fine Books, Connecticut, 1927.

4 Bonanno, G., *The Other Side of Sadness: What the New Science of Bereavement Tells Us about Life after Loss.* Basic Books, New York, 2009.

5 Fredrickson, B., *Positivity.* Crown, New York, 2009.

6 Bartrim, K., McCarthy, B., McCartney, D., Grant, G., Desbrow, B., and Irwin, C., Three consecutive nights of sleep loss: Effects of morning caffeine consumption on subjective sleepiness/ alertness, reaction time and simulated driving performance. *Transportation Research Part F: Traffic Psychology and Behaviour*, 70 (2020).

7 Rebar, A. L., Stanton, R., Geard, D., Short, C., Duncan, M. J., and Vandelanotte, C., A meta-meta-analysis of the effect of physical activity on depression and anxiety in non-clinical adult populations. *Health Psychology Review*, 9:3 (2015), 366–78.

8 Teo, A. R., HwaJung Choi, Andrea, S. B., Valenstein, M., Newsom, J. T., Dobscha, S. K., and Zivin, K., Does mode of contact with different types of social relationships predict depression in older adults? evidence from a nationally representative survey. *Journal of the American Geriatrics Society*, 2015.

Chapter 2

1 Beck, J. S., *Cognitive Behavior Therapy: Basics and Beyond*, 2nd edn. The Guilford Press, New York, 2011.

2 Pinkola Estes, C., *Women Who Run with the Wolves*. Random House, New York, 1996.

3 https://web.stanford.edu/~wine/202/g-and-b.html

Chapter 3

1 Feldman Barrett, L., *How Emotions Are Made*. Macmillan, New York, 2017.

2 Feldman Barrett, L., Gross, J., Christensen, T. C., and Benvenuto, M., Emotion differentiation and regulation. *Cognition and Emotion*. 15(2001), 713–24.

3 Benson, H., *The Relaxation Response*. HarperTorch, New York, 1976.

4 Kanouse, D. E., and Hanson, L., Negativity in evaluations. In E. E. Jones, D. E. Kanouse, S. Valins, H. H. Kelley, R. E. Nisbett and B. Weiner (eds), *Attribution: Perceiving the Causes of Behaviour*. 47–62. General Learning Press, Morristown, NJ, 1972.

5 Dolan, R. J., Vuilleumier, P., Amygdala automaticity in emotional processing. *Annals of the New York Academy of Sciences*. 985(2003), 348–55.

6 Tolle, E., *The Power of Now: A Guide to Spiritual Enlightenment*. Namaste, Vancouver, 2004.

7 Fredrickson, B., *Positivity*. Crown, New York, 2009.

8 Emmons, R. A., The psychology of gratitude: an introduction. In R. A. Emmons and M. E. McCullough (eds), *Series in Affective science: The Psychology of Gratitude*. 3–16. Oxford University Press, Oxford, 2004.

9 Gross, J. J., *Handbook of Emotion Regulation*. Guilford Press, New York, 2007.

Chapter 4

1 Mehrabian, A., *Silent Messages*, 1st edn. Wadsworth, Belmont, CA, 1971.

2 Cooper, D., *A Little Light on the Spiritual Laws*. Mobius, New York, 2004.

Chapter 5

1 Barks, C., *The Soul of Rumi: A New Collection of Ecstatic Poems*. HarperOne, San Francisco, 2002.

Chapter 6

1 Myss, C., *The Language of Archetypes: Discover the Forces that Shape your Destiny*. Audiobook. Sounds True, 2006.

2 Tolle, E., *The Art of Presence*. Audiobook. Sounds True, 2007

3 https://www.myss.com/

Chapter 7

1 Mehrabian, A., *Silent Messages*, 1st edn. Wadsworth, Belmont, CA, 1971.

Chapter 8

1 James, W. *The Principles of Psychology*. Henry Holt, New York, 1890.

Chapter 9

1 Amara, H., *Warrior Goddess Training: Become the Woman You Are Meant to Be*. Hay House, Carlsbad, CA, 2016.

2 Beck, A., The past and the future of cognitive therapy. *Journal of Psychotherapy Practice and Research*, 6 (1997), 276–84.

3 Dilts, R., Grinder, J., Delozier, J., and Bandler, R., *Neuro-Linguistic Programming: Volume I: The Study of the Structure of Subjective Experience*. Meta Publications, Cupertino, CA, 1980.

4 McDonnell, D., *How to Communicate Basically Brilliantly with Patients*. Self-published, 2013.

Chapter 10

1 Kabat-Zinn, J., *Full Catastrophe Living: Using the Wisdom of Your Body and Mind to Face Stress, Pain, and Illness*, 1st edn. Dell Publishing, New York, 1990.

2 Zaccaro, A., Piarulli, A., Laurino, M., Garbella, E., Menicucci, D., Neri, B., and Gemignani, A., How breath-control can change

your life: A systematic review on psycho-physiological correlates of slow breathing. *Frontiers in Human Neuroscience*, 12 (2018), 353.

3 Benson, H., *The Relaxation Response*, HarperTorch, New York, 1976.

Chapter 11

1 Barbe, W. B., Swassing, R. H., and Milone, M. N., *Teaching through modality Strengths: Concepts Practices*. Zaner-Bloser, Columbus, OH, 1979.

2 Fleming, N. D., *The VARK Modalities*. vark-learn.com, 2014.

Chapter 12

1 Fredrickson, B. L., Cohn, M. A., Coffey, K. A., Pek, J., and Finkel, S. M., Open hearts build lives: Positive emotions, induced through loving-kindness meditation, build consequential personal resources. *Journal of Personality and Social Psychology*, 95 (2008), 1045–62.

2 Kok, B. E., Coffey, K. A., Cohn, M. A., Catalino, L. I., Vacharkulksemsuk, T., Algoe, S. B., Brantley, M., and Fredrickson, B. L., How positive emotions build physical health: Perceived positive social connections account for the upward spiral between positive emotions and vagal tone. *Psychological Science*, 24 (2013), 1123–32.

3 https://chopra.com

4 Horowitz, S., Health benefits of meditation. *Alternative and Complementary Therapies*, 16 (2010), 223–8.; Chan, D., and Woollacott M., Effects of level of meditation experience on attentional focus: Is the efficiency of executive or orientation networks improved? *Journal of Alternative and Complementary Medicine*, 13 (2007), 651–7; Burns, J. L., Lee, R. M., and Brown, L. J., The effect of meditation on self-reported measures of stress, anxiety, depression, and perfectionism in a college population. *Journal of College Student Psychotherapy*, 25 (2011), 132–44.

5 Luberto, C. M., Shinday, N., Song, R., Philpotts, L. L., Park, E. R., Fricchione, G. L., and Yeh, G. Y., A systematic review and

meta-analysis of the effects of meditation on empathy, compassion, and prosocial behaviors. *Mindfulness*, 9:3 (2017), 708–24.

5 May, C. J., Ostafin, B. D., and Snippe, E., The relative impact of 15-minutes of meditation compared to a day of vacation in daily life: An exploratory analysis. *The Journal of Positive Psychology*, 15:2 (2020), 278–84.

7 Schlosser, M., Sparby, T., Vörös, S., Jones, R., and Marchant, N. L., Unpleasant meditation-related experiences in regular meditators: Prevalence, predictors, and conceptual considerations. *PLOS ONE*, 14:5 (2019), e0216643.

Chapter 13

1 Kabat-Zinn, J., *The Healing Power of Mindfulness: A New Way of Being*. Barnes & Noble, New York, 2018.

2 Tolle, E., *The Power of Now: A Guide to Spiritual Enlightenment*. Namaste, Vancouver, 2004.

3 https://www.nsf.gov/

4 https://heatherplett.com/2015/03/hold-space/

5 Shian-Ling Keng, Smoski, M. J., and Robins, C. J., Effects of mindfulness on psychological health: A review of empirical studies. *Clinical Psychology Review*, 31:6 (2011), 1041–56.

6 Gu, J., Strauss, C., Bond, R., and Cavanagh, K., How do mindfulness-based cognitive therapy and mindfulness-based stress reduction improve mental health and wellbeing? A systematic review and meta-analysis of meditation studies: Corrigendum. *Clinical Psychology Review*, 49 (2016), 119.

7 Jordan, C. H., Wan Wang, Donatoni, L., and Meier, B. P., Mindful eating: Trait and state mindfulness predict healthier eating behaviour. *Personality and Individual Differences*, 2014. https://doi.org/10.1016/j.paid.2014.04.013

8 Olson, K. L., and Emery, C. F., Mindfulness and weight loss: A systematic review. *Psychosomatic Medicine*, 77:1 (2015): 59–67.

Chapter 14

1 Mitima-Verloop, H. B., Mooren, T. T. M., and Boelen, P. A., Facilitating grief: An exploration of the function of funerals and rituals in relation to grief reactions. *Death Studies*, 2019. DOI: 10.1080/07481187.2019.1686090

2 https://www.bbc.co.uk/music/articles/a84df289-9e08-4a47-86e6-b91b7d94293f

3 Nadal, R., and Carlin, J., *Rafa: My Story*. Sphere, London, 2012.

4 Fiese, B. H., Tomcho, T. J., Douglas, M., Josephs, K., Poltrock, S., and Baker, T., A review of 50 years of research on naturally occurring family routines and rituals: Cause for celebration? *Journal of Family Psychology by the American Psychological Association*, 16:4 (2002), 381–90.

5 Brooks, A. W., Schroeder, J., Risen, J. L., Gino, F., Galinsky, A. D., Norton, M. I., and Schweitzer, M. E., Don't stop believing: rituals improve performance by decreasing anxiety. *Organizational Behavior and Human Decision Processes*, 137 (2016), 71–85.

6 Hobson, N. M., Bonk, D., and Inzlicht, M., Rituals decrease the neural response to performance failure. *PeerJ*, 5 (2017), e3363.

7 Damisch, L., Stoberock, B., and Mussweiler, T., Keep your fingers crossed!: How superstition improves performance. *Psychological Science*, 21:7 (2010), 1014–20.

8 Kostovičová, L., The differential effects of good luck belief on cognitive performance in boys and girls. *Europe's Journal of Psychology*, 15:1 (2019), 108–19.

Chapter 15

1 Mumford, A., *Putting Learning Styles to Work. Action Learning at Work*. 121–35. Gower, Brookfield, VT, 1997.

2 Barbe, W. B., Swassing, R. H., and Milone, M. N., *Teaching through Modality Strengths: Concepts Practices*. Zaner-Bloser, Columbus, OH, 1979.

3 Harrington, C., Teach learning skills, not learning styles: We are ALL multi-sensory learners. Cengage Learning Blog, 2014.

4 Dubord, G., Part 8. Cognitive illusions. *Canadian Family Physician*, 57:7 (2011), 799–800.

5 Klein, K., Boals, A., Expressive writing can increase working memory capacity. *Journal of Experimental Psychology*, 3:139 (2001), 520–33.

6 Davidson, K., Schwartz, A. R., Sheffield, D., McCord, R. S., Lepore, S. J., & Gerin, W., Expressive writing and blood pressure. In S. J. Lepore and J. M. Smyth (eds), *The Writing Cure: How Expressive Writing Promotes Health and Emotional Well-being*. 17–30. American Psychological Association, Washington, DC, 2002.

7 Baikie, K. A., Wilhelm, K., Emotional and physical health benefits of expressive writing. *Advances in Psychiatric Treatment*, 11:5 (2005), 338–46.

8 Smyth, J. M., Johnson, J. A., Auer, B. J., Lehman, E., Talamo, G., and Sciamanna, C. N., Online positive affect journaling in the improvement of mental distress and well-being in general medical patients with elevated anxiety symptoms: A preliminary randomized controlled trial. *JMIR Mental Health*, 5:4 (2018), e11290.

9 Karkou, V., Aithal, S., Zubala, A., and Meekums, B., Effectiveness of dance movement therapy in the treatment of adults with depression: A systematic review with meta-analyses. *Frontiers in Psychology*, 10 (2019), 936.

10 Leubner, D., and Hinterberger, T., Reviewing the effectiveness of music interventions in treating depression. *Frontiers in Psychology*, 8 (2017), 1109.

11 Wang, S., Mak, H. W., and Fancourt, D. Arts, mental distress, mental health functioning and life satisfaction: Fixed-effects analyses of a nationally-representative panel study. *BMC Public Health*, 20 (2020), 208.

Chapter 19

1 Lewis, D., *I Close My Eyes and See*. Findhorn Press, Moray, Scotland, 1996.

Chapter 20

1 Hunter, M. E., *Creative Scripts for Hypnotherapy*. Routledge, Oxon, 1994.

2 Cheek, D., *Hypnosis: The Application of Ideomotor Techniques*. Allyn & Bacon, Boston, MA, 1995.

3 Watts, T., *Crucial! Fantastic Inductions and Deepeners for the Professional Hypnotherapist*. Kindle edition, 2011.

4 Miller, G. A., The magical number seven, plus or minus two: Some limits on our capacity for processing information. *Psychological Review*, 63 (1956), 81–97.

Chapter 21

1 Covey, S. R., *The 7 Habits of Highly Effective People*. Simon & Schuster, New York, 2020.

2 https://www.mindtools.com/pages/article/newHTE_95.htm

3 Dubord, G., Part 8. Cognitive illusions. *Canadian Family Physician*, 57:7 (2011), 799–800.

4 Bandler, R., and Grinder, J., *Frogs into Princes: Introduction to Neurolinguistic Programming*. Eden Grove, 1990.

5 Carney, D. R., Cuddy, A. J. C., and Yap, A. J., Power posing: Brief nonverbal displays affect neuroendocrine levels and risk tolerance. *Psychological Science*, 21:10 (2010), 1363–8.

6 Dubord, G., Part 8. Cognitive illusions. *Canadian Family Physician*, 57:7 (2011), 799–800.

Index